Monika Hackl

Completeness Estimation of Austrian Cancer Incidence Data

Monika Hackl

Completeness Estimation of Austrian Cancer Incidence Data

Südwestdeutscher Verlag für Hochschulschriften

Impressum / Imprint
Bibliografische Information der Deutschen Nationalbibliothek: Die Deutsche Nationalbibliothek verzeichnet diese Publikation in der Deutschen Nationalbibliografie; detaillierte bibliografische Daten sind im Internet über http://dnb.d-nb.de abrufbar.
Alle in diesem Buch genannten Marken und Produktnamen unterliegen warenzeichen-, marken- oder patentrechtlichem Schutz bzw. sind Warenzeichen oder eingetragene Warenzeichen der jeweiligen Inhaber. Die Wiedergabe von Marken, Produktnamen, Gebrauchsnamen, Handelsnamen, Warenbezeichnungen u.s.w. in diesem Werk berechtigt auch ohne besondere Kennzeichnung nicht zu der Annahme, dass solche Namen im Sinne der Warenzeichen- und Markenschutzgesetzgebung als frei zu betrachten wären und daher von jedermann benutzt werden dürften.

Bibliographic information published by the Deutsche Nationalbibliothek: The Deutsche Nationalbibliothek lists this publication in the Deutsche Nationalbibliografie; detailed bibliographic data are available in the Internet at http://dnb.d-nb.de.
Any brand names and product names mentioned in this book are subject to trademark, brand or patent protection and are trademarks or registered trademarks of their respective holders. The use of brand names, product names, common names, trade names, product descriptions etc. even without a particular marking in this works is in no way to be construed to mean that such names may be regarded as unrestricted in respect of trademark and brand protection legislation and could thus be used by anyone.

Coverbild / Cover image: www.ingimage.com

Verlag / Publisher:
Südwestdeutscher Verlag für Hochschulschriften
ist ein Imprint der / is a trademark of
OmniScriptum GmbH & Co. KG
Heinrich-Böcking-Str. 6-8, 66121 Saarbrücken, Deutschland / Germany
Email: info@svh-verlag.de

Herstellung: siehe letzte Seite /
Printed at: see last page
ISBN: 978-3-8381-3868-8

Zugl. / Approved by: Wien, Medizinische Universität Wien, Diss., 2013

Copyright © 2014 OmniScriptum GmbH & Co. KG
Alle Rechte vorbehalten. / All rights reserved. Saarbrücken 2014

Mama † 2007

Contents

Acknowledgements 5
Abstract 7
Zusammenfassung 9
1 Introduction **11**
1.1 The Austrian National Cancer Registry 11
1.2 International accreditation of the Austrian National Cancer Registry 12
1.3 Cancer registry goes statistics 13
1.4 Cancer statistics for decision-making: How sound are Austrian's cancer registry data? 14
    1.4.1 Cases registered & Population covered 14
    1.4.2 Incidence 15
    1.4.3 Prevalence 17
    1.4.4 Survival 18
    1.4.5 Mortality 20
1.5 Comparability of population-based cancer data 22
    1.5.1 "Completeness of registration" vs. "Completeness of case ascertainment" 22
    1.5.2 Completeness of case ascertainment as a basic quality criterion for cancer registries 23
1.6 Objectives of the study 23

2 Material and Methods **25**
2.1 Database 25
2.2 International recognized methods to estimate completeness of case ascertainment 25
    2.2.1 Stability of incidence rates over time 29
    2.2.2 Comparison of incidence rates in different populations 29
    2.2.3 Shape of age-specific curves 30
    2.2.4 Incidence rates of childhood cancers 31
    2.2.5 Mortality:Incidence ratio 32
    2.2.6 Number of sources/notifications per case 33
    2.2.7 Histological verification of diagnosis 34
    2.2.8 Re-screening of already used sources 36
    2.2.9 Independent case ascertainment - Hospital-Discharge-Only 37

  2.2.10 Capture–recapture methods 38
  2.2.11 Death certificate methods - DCN/M:I method.........................40
  2.2.12 Death certificate methods - The Flow Method........................42
2.3 Definitions 44
  2.3.1 Tumor entities 44
  2.3.2 Age-adjustment..45
  2.3.3 Test of significance 46

3 Results by findings 47

3.1 Time series 47
3.2 Regional pattern..51
3.3 Tumor sites 56

4 Discussion..61

4.1 Evaluation of methods..61
  4.1.1 Evaluation of Stability of incidence rates over time, Comparison of incidence rates in different populations 61
  4.1.2 Evaluation of Mortality:Incidence ratio.....................................62
  4.1.3 Evaluation of the Flow Method 63
  4.1.4 Evaluation of the concept of Hospital-Discharge-Only (HDO) ..64
4.2 Further Perspectives 65
  4.2.1 Retain already established analyses and strengthen standardized routine jobs...65
  4.2.2 Investigate the Flow Method 66
  4.2.3 Enhance the concept of Hospital-Discharge-Only (HDO).........68
4.3 Strengths and limitations of this study 71

5 Conclusion 74

6 References..78

7 Glossar 86

Acknowledgements

First of all I want to thank my colleagues and the head of my department at Statistics Austria for making this thesis possible, for supporting and challenging me. Thanks to my national and international colleagues and friends in the field of cancer registration and cancer statistics for many lively and fruitful discussions.

Also a special thanks to my supervisor and the doctoral thesis committee for supporting me to investigate the completeness of case ascertainment of the Austrian National Cancer Registry data.

Last but not least I want to thank my family for always believing in me. Part of the time I used to work at my thesis was actual their time. Thanks for giving it to me and for all your patience with me!

Abstract

Background: Meaningful regional comparisons of cancer incidence and further analysis (e.g. comparison of survival rates) are only possible if completeness of case ascertainment is assessed to be approximately the same for all regions or it is indicated which allows for corrections in order to establish comparable data. The aim of the study is to evaluate internationally recommended methods for completeness estimation in cancer registries.

Methods: Five of these methods applicable to the Austrian National Cancer Registry (ANCR) and suitable for routine use have been evaluated: Stability of incidence rates over time, Comparison of incidence rates in different populations, Mortality:Incidence ratio (M:I ratio), Flow Method and Hospital-Discharge-Only (HDO) index. Cancer incidence data, data from causes of death statistics and data from hospital discharge statistics were used to estimate the completeness of the ANCR on national and on regional level.

Results: With exception of the Flow Method's regional analyses, all results show the same pattern of completeness. Two major assumptions could be verified: First, data for federal states showing higher incidence rates are more complete than data for federal states showing lower incidence rates. The benefits of a regional cancer registry – i.e. smaller population covered and geographical proximity – improve data quality only if they are combined with outstanding personal commitment. Second, ANCR's data show lower incidence rates in the most recent years because completeness is lower in these years.

Conclusion: These results seem to be reliable because different concepts for completeness estimation show equivalent results. Analysis showed that the Flow Method was not appropriate for the ANCR under current conditions and that the HDO index was biased due to lack of unique personal identifiers. Further investigations on the Flow Method and on the HDO index are recommended to gain a valid estimator of completeness.

Zusammenfassung

Hintergrund: Sinnvolle regionale Vergleiche der Krebsinzidenz und weiterer Analysen (wie z.B. der Überlebenswahrscheinlichkeit) sind nur möglich wenn die Vollzähligkeit der Daten entweder für alle Regionen als in etwa gleich angenommen werden kann oder wenn eine nummerische Vollzähligkeitsschätzung die Erstellung vergleichbarer Datenbestände ermöglicht. Ziel dieser Studie ist international empfohlene Methoden zur Vollzähligkeitsschätzung von Krebsregistern zu evaluieren.

Methode: Fünf der für das Österreichische Krebsregister (Austrian National Cancer Registry, ANCR) anwendbaren Methoden, die auch im Routinebetrieb einsetzbar sind, wurden evaluiert: Stabilität im Zeitverlauf, Vergleich der Inzidenzraten in verschiedenen Populationen, Mortalität/Inzidenz-Ratio (M/I-Ratio), Flow Methode, Hospital-Discharge-Only (HDO) Index. Es wurden Daten aus dem Krebsregister, der Todesursachenstatistik und der Spitalsentlassungsstatistik verwendet, um die Vollzähligkeit des ANCR auf nationaler und regionaler Ebene zu beurteilen.

Ergebnis: Mit Ausnahme der regionalen Ergebnisse der Flow Methode, lieferten alle Methoden das gleiche Muster der Vollzähligkeit. Folgende zwei Hauptannahmen konnten bestätigt werden: Erstens, die Daten der Bundesländer mit höheren Krebsinzidenzraten sind im Allgemeinen vollzähliger als die Daten von Bundesländern mit niedrigeren Krebsinzidenzraten. Die Vorteile eines regionalen Krebsregisters – wie z.B. eine kleinere Grundbevölkerung und die räumliche Nähe – wirken sich nur dann positiv auf die Datenqualität aus, wenn sie mit außerordentlichem persönlichem Engagement kombiniert sind. Zweitens, die niedrigeren

Inzidenzraten des ANCR für die jüngsten veröffentlichten Diagnosejahre sind auf eine niedrigere Vollzähligkeit der Daten in diesen Jahren zurückzuführen.

Diskussion: Diese Ergebnisse scheinen zuverlässig, da verschiedene Konzepte der Vollzähligkeitsschätzung zu gleichen Ergebnissen führten. Die Analyse zeigte, dass die Flow Methode unter den derzeitigen Bedingungen nicht für das ANCR geeignet ist, und dass der HDO Index durch das Fehlen eines eindeutigen Personenkennzeichens verfälscht ist. Um gültige Vollzähligkeitsschätzer zu erhalten, werden weitere Untersuchungen zur Flow Methode und zum HDO Index empfohlen.

1 Introduction

1.1 The Austrian National Cancer Registry

The Austrian National Cancer Registry operated by the National Statistical Office, Statistics Austria, is a population based cancer registry with a clear epidemiological background. It is an important data source for health policy, for health reporting, and for scientific research. Cancer statistics resulting from this registry provide data on cancer incidence, survival and prevalence, stratified by various demographic and tumor specific parameters. Data on cancer mortality are based on the causes of death statistics, also prepared by Statistics Austria. Data based on cancer incidence and cancer mortality are available for the whole Austrian population with the possibility of regional analyses based on the municipality identifier (Statistik Austria: Dokumentation „Krebsstatistik", 2011).

The Austrian National Cancer Registry can look back on a long-standing tradition. Since more than 50 years the cancer registry has been operating, for quite a long time based on legal regulations. The Cancer Statistics Act (Krebsstatistikgesetz, 1969) was already established in 1969 and regulates data collection and persons and institutions obliged to notify. Subjects of data collection are tumor type, tumor site, progress of the disease and personal patient data. The Cancer Statistics Ordinance was added to the Cancer Statistics Act in 1978 (Krebsstatistikverordnung, 1978). It regulates the notification date and frequency as well as the notifiable data in detail and presents the notification form.

To assure data quality and international comparability of the Austrian National Cancer Registry data, data collection as well as data processing follow closely international recommendations developed by the European Network of Cancer Registries (ENCR) and the International Association of Cancer Registries (IACR). These recommendations supported by the International Agency for Research on Cancer (IARC) deal mainly with data collection characteristics, set a frame for tumors to be documented and provide definitions (e.g. for date of diagnosis, basis of diagnosis, extent of disease at the time of diagnosis) and plausibility checks (like cross-checking of tumor site and histology). Recommended rules concerning the classification of multiple primaries are implemented in the Austrian National Cancer Registry as well.

To assure completeness of case ascertainment and hence regional and international comparability, checks on completeness are performed to test compliance with law. Statistics Austria regularly provides quality indicators and indirect measures for completeness (Statistik Austria, 2012). These indicators give a general overview of the registry´s quality but do not allow a reliable assessment of completeness.

However, possibilities to monitor compliance with the obligation to notify cancer cases are limited. Statistics Austria therefore estimates expected numbers of notifiable tumors according to hospital size and main points of treatment based on the number of notified tumors in the previous years. If fewer tumor notifications are forwarded than expected, Statistics Austria reminds the hospitals of their obligation to notify each cancer case (Statistik Austria: Dokumentation „Krebsstatistik", 2011).

1.2 International accreditation of the Austrian National Cancer Registry

Publication of the Austrian Cancer Incidence data through the International Agency for Research on Cancer (IARC) confirms high quality of the data. The

IARC is part of the World Health Organization (WHO), situated in Lyon, France. The agencies focus is on research on causes of cancer and mechanisms of carcinogenesis in humans as well as on the development of scientific strategies for cancer control. In these fields epidemiological and laboratory research is conducted. A basic reference for international epidemiological cancer research is the publication "Cancer Incidence in Five Continents". This definitive book provides worldwide data on cancer incidence. The acceptance of a registries' data for this publication is regarded as a seal of approval.

In an international context there are few epidemiological cancer registries covering a comparable or greater population. Compared to the 100 European cancer registries whose data were accepted by IARC for publication in Cancer Incidence in Five Continents, (Curado et al., 2007), the Austrian National Cancer Registry covers the seventh largest area as well as the seventh largest population. Only 27 out of the 100 cancer registries work on a legal basis prescribing an obligation of notification.

1.3 Cancer registry goes statistics

Medical documentation by itself is no registry, a registry is no statistic and a (frequency-) statistic is no analysis. However, one is a follow-up to the other. Austrian cancer statistics are the output of the data of the Austrian National Cancer Registry operated by Statistics Austria. While cancer statistics are publicly available and accessible, the registry operates virtually unnoticed by the general public.

The information stored in the cancer registry is compiled according to various rules. Each cancer notification form adds some information to the consistent database. A snapshot of the database is preserved once a year. This snapshot is called the authentic data set. The authentic data set is the basis for cancer statistics and all further analysis. Based on this data set Statistics Austria generates the tables for e.g. the yearbook of health statistics and for its website. These published data are easily accessible and may be used free of charge.

1.4 Cancer statistics for decision-making: How sound are Austrian's cancer registry data?

1.4.1 Cases registered & Population covered

The comparability of cancer key figures depends primarily on the type of cases covered by registration and the criteria for inclusion in the published statistics. Correct and reproducible classification and coding as well as the method of follow-up are criteria for comparability. Furthermore, it is necessary to have demographic key figures for the population covered by the registry.

The Austrian National Cancer Registry documents all diagnosed cancer cases, whether they are in-situ or invasive tumors. The fact that only primary malignancies are registered means that multiple tumors are counted as two or more tumors while metastases and recurrences are not yet registered. Cancer cases that come to the attendance of the cancer registry by Death-Certificate-Only (DCO cases) are included in the cancer statistics. Cancer incidence numbers (comprising only invasive malignancies), are published excluding in-situ cases and non-melanoma skin cancer. This is a common strategy as non-melanoma skin cancer is often diagnosed outside hospitals and the completeness of case ascertainment shows remarkable differences between cancer registries. Currently, the Austrian National Cancer Registry uses the International Classification of Diseases for Oncology in its third version (ICD-O-3, 2000). When the registry changed to version three all cases in the registry were recoded. For this purpose a tool developed by IARC was used, no text review or chart review was done. Follow-up is conducted passively, when cancer notification forms stating the death of a person or death certificates are received as well actively, using the central population registry for selected cases. The Austrian National Cancer Registry covers the whole Austrian residential population. For four out of the nine federal states (Vorarlberg, Tyrol, Carinthia and Salzburg) data are collected via a regional cancer registry. All demographic indicators needed are provided by Statistics Austria, being the national statistical institute.

1.4.2 Incidence

Cancer incidence is defined as the number of new cancer cases occurring in a specified population during a defined period of time, usually a year. Cancer incidence can be calculated per cancer site, stage, sex, age or region. The cancer incidence rate is expressed as the number of cancer cases per 100,000 population at risk. For cancer sites that occur in only one sex, the sex-specific population (e.g. females for cervical cancer) is used.

Age-specific and age-adjusted (age-standardized) incidence rates are published on a routine basis. The direct age-adjusted incidence rate is a weighted average of the age-specific rates, with weights being the proportions of persons in the corresponding age group of the standard population. The potential confounding effect of a population's age structure is eliminated by using age-adjusted rates for comparisons across different regions or time spans.

Each calendar year about 38,000 malignant invasive tumors are diagnosed in Austria. Since 1996 men are confronted with a cancer diagnosis more often the women. One reason for this trend is the increasing number of prostate cancer diagnoses. Prostate cancer has been the most frequent cancer site in men since 1994; with 4,488 cases diagnosed in 2010 (age adjusted 60.0 cases per 100,000 men, adjusted for world standard population, Segi, 1960). In former days lung cancer was the most common cancer diagnosis in men, now ranging on the second position, followed by colon cancer. Breast cancer has always been the most frequent cancer site in women with 5,105 cases or age adjusted 64.9 cases per 100,000 women in 2010 (Statistik Austria, 2013). Comparison of incidence rates across federal states shows rather large differences. It seems that federal states with data provided by a regional registry show higher cancer incidence rates, probably because their data are more complete than those of federal states without a regional registry (Figure 1). While the mean Austrian age adjusted incidence rate for all malignant tumors for the years of diagnosis 2001 to 2010 is approximately 256/100,000, clearly higher rates are found in Carinthia and Tyrol (293 and 291) contrasted to lower rates in Styria, Lower Austria, and Vienna (250, 245 and 244, respectively) (Statistik Austria, 2013, own calculations).

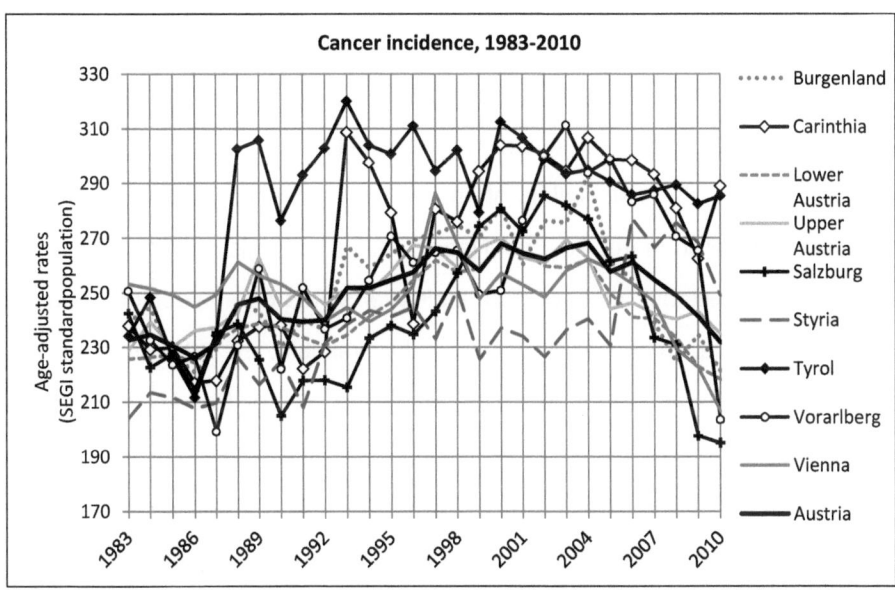

Figure 1: Age-adjusted incidence rate for all malignant tumors, Austria and federal states, 1983-2010 (per 24.09.2012)

1.4.3 Prevalence

The number of all cancer patients alive in a defined population on a certain date is called cancer prevalence. In contrast to incidence, overall prevalence is not dependent on the time of diagnosis. Every patient once diagnosed with cancer is a part of the prevalent cancer patient group. Although the data of diagnosis is not needed to calculate overall prevalence, it is relevant for stratified prevalence. For health care planning and care research not only the total number of living cancer patients is of interest. For example, for resource allocation in acute cancer care the number of patients diagnosed during the last two years is relevant. For other fields of health planning, e.g. the number of so called cancer survivors is necessary. This means the number of patients with a cancer diagnose a defined time span ago. Estimates on cancer prevalence can not only be stratified by time span since diagnosis, but also by sex, tumor site or other characteristics such as age or region. So far prevalence has not been calculated at regional level.

The bases for the calculation of the Austrian cancer prevalence are all patients registered in the Austrian National Cancer Registry (Zielonke, 2011). For all those patients a follow-up of their vital status on a specified reference day is available. In the analysis currently available, all patients diagnosed between 1983 and 2011 and still alive on the 31st of December 2011 are included.

At the end of the year 2011 303,761 persons with a prior cancer diagnosis were alive, thereof 160,079 women and 143,710 men. In other words, 36 out of 1,000 Austrian residents were alive with a cancer diagnosis at this point of time. The biggest fraction of women living with cancer was those of breast cancer patients (64,560), followed by women diagnosed with cancer of the uterus (21,312) and cancer of the colon (18,537). The most frequent tumor site for men living with cancer was prostate cancer (55,072), followed by cancer of the colon (21,016) and the bladder (11,522).

1.4.4 Survival

Relative survival – the ratio of the observed survival to the survival expected in the general population of same age and sex – is calculated by Statistics Austria in order to eliminate the effect of competing causes of mortality. For the calculation of relative survival, the life table method was used to estimate observed survival and Ederer II to estimate expected survival (Ederer, 1961). Calendar year-, sex- and age-specific life tables also provided by Statistics Austria were used. Calculations were conducted using SAS 9.3. The bases for the analysis program were SAS macros provided by Paul Dickman

(Dickman, 2013). According to the latest international development, multiple primaries were included (Concord study, 2013).

Several methodological limitations like lead-time bias, length time bias or over-diagnosis can influence survival probabilities. These limitations bias survival time as they add days, weeks or even months of survival without postponing the date of death. Furthermore, survival analyses are no substitute for the assessment of quality of live.

Nevertheless, 5-year cumulative relative survival is a common measure for survival probabilities. It puts the survival probability of the cancer patients in relation to the survival probability of the general population. The survival probability of the general population is set to 100% and survival probability of the cancer patients is expressed as proportion. The 5-year cumulative relative survival for cancer patients diagnosed in 2006 was 61%, 60% for men and 63% for women (Statistik Austria, 2013). Compared to international cancer survival statistics results and trends are reasonable. Overall cancer survival is related strongly to the cancer site and the stage at diagnosis. Age and sex are also seen as a strong outcome predictor (Berrino, 2007).

Clearly different survival rates are seen when 5-year cumulative relative survival for all tumor sites are compared across federal states. As almost equal survival rates can be expected for all regions, reasons explaining the differences are to be investigated. Different quality of follow-up cannot explain the differences as it is done centrally for all federal states in the same manner. Differences in overall survival could be caused by the case mix although the exclusion of prostate cancer which is the most likely explanation does not change the pattern of survival rates across the federal states. Nevertheless, screening and overdiagnosis are possible explanations and it should be looked at regional screening pattern for various tumor entities.

Another explanation implies that different levels of completeness of case ascertainment across the federal states bias survival rates. Data were pooled (2004-2006) to compensate for random variation (Figure 2).

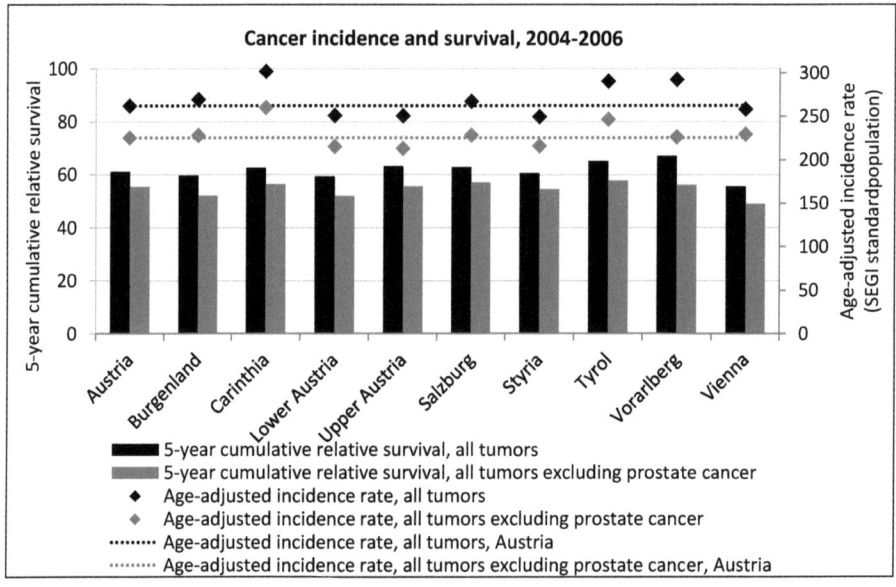

Figure 2: Austrian age adjusted incidence and survival rates for all malignant tumors and all malignant tumors excluding prostate cancer, 2004-2006 (per 24.09.2012)

1.4.5 Mortality

Causes of death statistics have a long standing tradition in many countries. This is also true for Austria, where causes of death statistics date back to the 19th century. Statistics on mortality are often used as a proxy for health statistics as they provide information on the underlying disease. Available data draw a picture of the health status of a population and are often used for clinical studies.

Cancer was the underlying cause of death for 19,992 persons (26%) in the year 2011. Almost 20% of all cancer deaths were caused by lung cancer, followed by colon cancer (slightly over 10%), cancer of the blood and blood-forming organs, pancreas and breast (each below 10%).

Age adjusted mortality rates for all malignant tumors also vary across the federal states but do not show the same regional pattern as incidence data. Data in figure 3 are shown for three years combined. Data were pooled to reduce random variation. Data for 2004 to 2006 are shown, as these are the latest years to calculate five year survival. Data for 2008-2010 are shown as these are the latest data available for cancer incidence. Mortality rates declined for each federal state, Salzburg and Tyrol constantly show the lowest mortality rates and Vienna the highest.

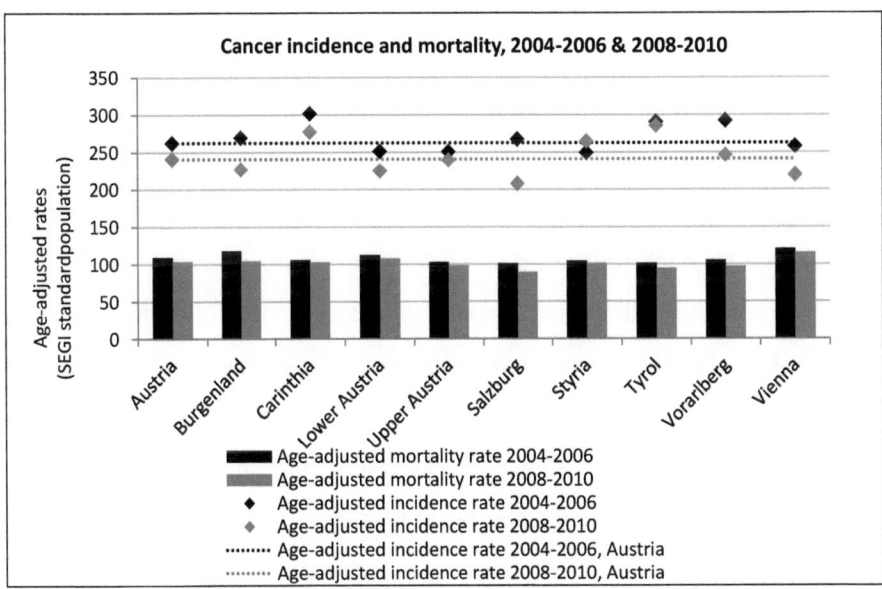

Figure 3: Austrian age adjusted incidence and mortality rates for all malignant tumors, Austria and federal states, 2004-2006 & 2008-2010 (per 24.09.2012)

1.5 Comparability of population-based cancer data

Comparability of cancer key figures depends not only on the availability of correct definitions as discussed in the epidemiological chapter "Cases registered & population covered" but also on the completeness of the registry.

1.5.1 "Completeness of registration" vs. "Completeness of case ascertainment"

For the discussion of completeness of cancer registration two different dimensions of completeness have to be considered: One dimension of completeness is referred to as "Completeness of registration", the other dimension as "Completeness of case ascertainment". These concepts are translated into German using "Vollständigkeit" and "Vollzähligkeit", respectively (Mattauch, Lehnert, Krieg and Hense (2003).

Completeness of registration refers to each single variable documented in the cancer registry. A completeness of 100% describing the variable "gender" means that for each registered person his or her sex is known. As for each variable recorded in the cancer registry the total number of registrations and the number of missing cases is known, completeness of registration can be easily calculated.

Completeness of case ascertainment specifies the number of cancer cases that are documented in the cancer registry as a proportion of all cancer cases diagnosed, usually published per year of diagnosis. As the absolute number of all cancer cases diagnosed within one calendar year is not known – to estimate this number is the task of the cancer registry - it is only possible to use various methods to estimate the completeness of case ascertainment for a registry.

1.5.2 Completeness of case ascertainment as a basic quality criterion for cancer registries

Quality and international comparability of cancer incidence and other key figures based on cancer registry data depend strongly on the completeness of case ascertainment of the registry. Therefore registration of the greatest possible number of cancer cases is the very first aim of every population based cancer registry. When interpreting cancer incidence rates and survival or prevalence estimates checks on completeness are important in order to distinguish between different regional risk, different regional distribution of tumor sites and different regional completeness of case ascertainment.

As the real number of new cancer cases occurring during a year is not known, the absolute number of cancer cases as well as the completeness of the cancer registry can only be estimated. Parkin and Bray (2009) provide an internationally recognized overview of different methods for completeness estimation. Qualitative methods evaluate completeness in relation to other registries or comparing different time spans whereas quantitative methods provide a numerical estimator for completeness.

1.6 Objectives of the study

The aim of the study is to evaluate internationally recommended methods for completeness estimation in cancer registries as meaningful regional comparisons of cancer incidence and all further analysis (e.g. comparison of survival rates) are only possible if the completeness of case ascertainment is known. Either the completeness is approximately the same for all compared regions or completeness is expressed as a specific figure so that cancer incidence and all related parameters can be corrected in order to establish comparable data.

First various internationally recommended methods will be described briefly and analyzed in respect for the applicability of the method for the Austrian National Cancer Registry and the possibility of implementing it into a routine workflow.

Second a subset of the described methods will be used to estimate the completeness of case ascertainment of the Austrian National Cancer Registry on national and regional level. The validity of the results will be assessed afterwards, comparing the results of the selected methods.

The study's findings shall be used to develop a meaningful instrument for completeness estimation out of the repertoire of applicable methods to enable further investigation to estimate precise and valid figures for the completeness of case ascertainment on a national level and for each federal state and to extrapolate cancer incidence data equivalent to a 100% complete data base.

2 Material and Methods

2.1 Database

For this study data from the Austrian National Cancer Registry, from the causes of death statistics and from the hospital discharge statistics were used. See "Statistik Austria: Dokumentation „Krebsstatistik", (2011), "Statistik Austria: Statistik der Standesfälle einschließlich Todesursachenstatistik ab 2010", (2012) and "Statistik Austria: Dokumentation "Spitalsentlassungsstatistik ab 1989", (2012).

2.2 International recognized methods to estimate completeness of case ascertainment

A standard work for many cancer registries is "Cancer Registration: Principles and Methods" by Jensen, Parkin, MacLennan, Muir and Skeet (1991). The chapter "Quality and Quality Control" discusses the estimation of completeness of cancer registration in a rather basic manner. It is stated that the assessment of completeness should be constantly monitored and that many of the checks described in the chapter should be implemented in the registries´ computer systems. For checks on completeness it is recommended to monitor the proportions of death certificates received for which no registration has previously been made as a part of all registrations and to compare the data from the latest incidence year with those of previous years on a site-specific basis.

These days literature distinguishes between DCN and DCO cases. For death-certificate-notified cases (DCN) usually hospitals or the certifying physician are contacted to gather further information. If further information is obtained, the case is registered. A death-certificate-only case (DCO) is a cancer case which comes to the attention of the cancer registry only because of the death certificate. Primarily registration and trace-back failed. Interpreting the DCO index one should bear in mind that it is not sensitive to cancers which have low case fatality rates. For cancers with high lethality the index is higher than for cancers with a better prognosis, independent of the level of completeness of case ascertainment. The informative value therefore depends stronger on the site-specific survival than on completeness (Brenner, 1995). For tumor sites with a good prognosis cases are not that rapidly reported via death certificate resulting in a low DCO index for this site but nevertheless the cases are missing. For long term survivors the cancer can even fail to be the underlying cause of death. However, every strong break in time series should alert the cancer registry experts. As no information concerning tumor morphology, tumor stage or date of diagnosis is available for DCO cases, these cases cause validity problems anyway.

Three years after "Cancer Registration: Principles and Methods" by Jensen, et al. (1991), the technical report "Comparability and Quality in Cancer Registration" was released by IARC (Parkin, Chen, Ferlay, Galceran, Storm and Whealan, 1994). Comparability, completeness and validity are the main topics of the report. The methods of completeness estimation for cancer registration are summarized under three headings: data sources, independent case ascertainment and historic data method. Methods of these categories are listed in table 1 (the structure of table 1 follows basically the structure of Parkin and Bray (2009)).

In 2009 Parkin and Bray published two papers to update the 1994 report. The paper dealing with completeness of case ascertainment categorizes the methods already described in 1994 into two groups. Qualitative (or semi-quantitative) methods use other registries or time spans as references and give only an indication of the degree of completeness. Quantitative methods provide a numerical estimator for completeness.

The Flow Method (Bullard, Coleman, Robinson, Lutz, Bell, Peto, 2000) is added to the methods of 1994 and the Death Certificate Method is described in a more comprehensible way. Table 1 gives an overview of possible methods for estimating the completeness of case ascertainment integrating the 1994 ideas and the 2009 structure of qualitative and quantitative methods. Subsequent to table 1, all methods introduced are described and their applicability to the Austrian National Cancer Registry as well as their suitability for routine use are assessed. Reasons for inclusion/non-inclusion into the study are discussed.

Table 1: Overview of possible methods estimating the completeness of case ascertainment comparing Parkin et al. (1994) and Parkin and Bray (2009).

1994 \ 2009	Qualitative Methods	Quantitative Methods
Historic Data Methods	(1) Stability of incidence rates over time (2) Comparison of incidence rates in different populations (3) Shape of age-specific curves (4) Incidence rates of childhood cancers	
Independent Case Ascertainment	(5) Mortality:Incidence ratio	(8) Re-screening of already used sources (9) Using data sets compiled independently of the cancer registry's case-finding proccdures – e.g. hospital discharge data (10) Capture–recapture methods
Independent Data Sets	(6) Number of sources/notifications per case (7) Histological verification of diagnosis	Death certificate methods: (11) DCN/M:I Method
Not established in 1994		Death certificate methods: (12) The Flow Method

2.2.1 Stability of incidence rates over time

Brief description

Incidence rates for recent data are compared with those from the same registry in earlier periods. Comparisons are conducted either within age groups or using a method for age-adjustment.

Applicability to the Austrian National Cancer Registry

Applicability is given, as absolute incidence figures and age-adjusted incidence rates have been available since 1983 on national and regional level.

Suitability for routine use

Suitability is given, as trends can be evaluated easily using available data.

Reasons for inclusion/non-inclusion into the study

This method was included into the study to establish a basic overview of the available cancer data. Absolute incidence figures and age-adjusted incidence rates were analyzed for time trends on national and regional level. All analyses were conducted in a descriptive way only.

2.2.2 Comparison of incidence rates in different populations

Brief description

Time trends are compared with results from similar populations within the registry or with demographically comparable populations elsewhere. Differences between regions may reflect specific local variations in prevalence of risk factors or the presence or intensity of screening for some cancers. However, systematic discrepancies (across several sites) provide evidence of possible under- or over-registration.

Applicability to the Austrian National Cancer Registry

Applicability is given, as absolute incidence figures and age-adjusted incidence rates have been available since 1983 on national and regional level.

Suitability for routine use

Suitability is given, as trends can be evaluated easily using available data.

Reasons for inclusion/non-inclusion into the study

This method was included into the study for gaining additional information to the results from "Stability of incidence rates over time". Absolute incidence figures, age-adjusted incidence rates and time trends were compared across federal states. All analyses were conducted in a descriptive way only.

2.2.3 Shape of age-specific curves

Brief description

For the most epithelial cancers incidence figures increase with age. Although a decline of incidence rates in the oldest age-groups is usual and could be caused by various factors, under-ascertainment must always be considered. However, not all cancer sites show the typical pattern of a monotone increase of log(incidence) with age.

Applicability to the Austrian National Cancer Registry

Applicability is given, as age-specific incidence curves can be calculated using available data.

Suitability for routine use

Suitability is given, as routine data can be used.

Reasons for inclusion/non-inclusion into the study

This method was not included into the study as it does not give a quick overview of completeness nor quantify completeness. Considering the time range of more than 30 years and the various cancer sites for Austria and for all federal states would exceed the scope of this work. Nevertheless, the method provides in-depth results about cancer sites deserving special emphasis in data collection. The method is therefore recommended for further investigation.

2.2.4 Incidence rates of childhood cancers

Brief description

With respect to childhood cancer, the incidence rates in the childhood age groups (0-4, 5-9, and 10-14 years) show much less variability than in adults although there are well-documented differences by geography or ethnicity for specific types of childhood cancer. The possibility of under-registration (or duplicate registration) in this age range can be investigated by comparing the observed age-specific rates with 'expected' rates in the childhood age range. The 'expected' rates, e.g. limiting values for the lowest and highest deciles, are published in CI5, Volume VIII (p67).

Applicability to the Austrian National Cancer Registry

Applicability is given, as childhood cancer is notifiable under Austrian law.

Suitability for routine use

Suitability is given, as routine data can be used.

Reasons for inclusion/non-inclusion into the study

This method was not included into the study as childhood cancer covers only a very specific part of cancer registration. It does not necessarily give information about the completeness of case ascertainment of the whole registry. Nevertheless, cancer incidence within the pediatric age range is highly interesting for the comparison of cancer incidence across the federal states and will be analyzed in the report of the Austrian National Cancer Registry on childhood cancer.

2.2.5 Mortality:Incidence ratio

Brief description

The Mortality:Incidence ratio (M:I ratio) is a comparison of the number of deaths, obtained from a source independent of the registry (usually, the vital statistics system), and the number of new cases of a specific cancer registered in the same period of time.

Applicability to the Austrian National Cancer Registry

Applicability is given, as causes of death statistics are available for the Austrian National Cancer Registry electronically.

Suitability for routine use

The method is widely-used but only of limited suitability for routine use unless equal survival rates for all regions under comparison can be assumed. Interpretation of M:I ratio is difficult, first no absolute reference values exist and second the M:I ratio is highly influenced by survival times. Although Parkin and Bray (2009) subsume the M:I ratio under the qualitative methods, many cancer registries use it for the estimation of expected incidence numbers assuming equal survival rates for all regions.

Reasons for (non-)inclusion into the study

This method was included into the study as Austrian mortality data are of good quality and high completeness of case ascertainment and therefore obviously can give valuable information on cancer incidence. M:I ratio was only used as a qualitative method as equal survival rates for all compared regions could not be assumed.

2.2.6 Number of sources/notifications per case

Brief description

The number of sources per case indicates the use of various routine case-finding procedures. Sources are for e.g. hospital patient disease information systems, pathology reports, radiotherapy notes or death certificates. The higher the average number of sources per case is, the higher will be the completeness of case ascertainment.

Applicability to the Austrian National Cancer Registry

The method could be applied as every cancer notification is stored in the cancer registry, including detailed information about the sender. Due to different registration procedures for federal states with or without regional cancer registry the number of sources is not meaningful. The number of notifications per case is not valid as well, as some hospitals send a cancer notification form only once and others send forms for every contact with the patient. In general, no reference values exist as the definition of "source" and the process of registration vary between cancer registries. Furthermore, the assumption that a higher number of sources per case results in higher completeness is only applicable to a limited extent.

Suitability for routine use

Basically, the method would be suitable for routine use as the necessary information is easily available.

Reasons for (non-)inclusion into the study

This method was not included into the study for reasons of applicability as described above.

2.2.7 Histological verification of diagnosis

Brief description

Histological verification, later broadened to morphological verification (including cytology), was primarily used as an indicator of validity, describing confidence in the diagnosis. The percentage of morphologically verified tumors depends strongly on tumor site, as not all sites are equally accessible for biopsy, and furthermore on the development of medical imaging. However, concerning completeness of case ascertainment a very high proportion of cases diagnosed by histology or cytology suggests over-reliance on the pathology laboratory as source of information and failure to find cases diagnosed by other means.

Applicability to the Austrian National Cancer Registry

This method can be applied to the Austrian data, as the method of tumor diagnosis is stored as a variable in the registry.

Suitability for routine use

The use of routine data and a very easy way of index calculation make the percentage of morphological verification (MV%) basically suitable for routine use. Interpretation of the MV% is not as easy as its calculation. The index is highly influenced by the percentage of DCO cases which is unproblematic if the index is used for quality control, as DCO cases are of low quality. For completeness control, DCO cases also reduce MV%. This reduction does not reflect a deficiency as DCO cases are known by causes of death statistics and added to the registry. Furthermore, different follow back procedures of DCO cases add an uncontrollable bias to the percentage of DCO cases and consequently to MV%.

Reasons for (non-)inclusion into the study

This method was not included into the study for reasons of index interpretation as described in "Suitability for routine use".

2.2.8 Re-screening of already used sources

Brief description

Using a protocol, all cases diagnosed or treated at one hospital during a defined period of time are checked to identify notifiable cancer cases. The established file of notifiable tumors and the cancer registry data are linked to provide the number of missing cases in the registry and to estimate under-registration.

Applicability to the Austrian National Cancer Registry

Basically the method would be applicable to the Austrian National Cancer Registry as cases gathered directly at hospital provide enough information on patient identification for record-linkage with the cancer registry. As differences concerning the notification of cancer cases between hospitals are likely, the method relying on data from only one hospital is not applicable to estimate the completeness of case ascertainment for the Austrian National Cancer Registry. The method could rather be used for auditing various hospitals on how conscientious they are about reporting cancer cases to the registry.

Suitability for routine use

This method is not suitable for routine use as the approach is very time-consuming and therefore disproportional expensive compared to the expected results.

Reasons for (non-)inclusion into the study

This method was not included into the study for reasons of applicability and suitability as described above.

2.2.9 Independent case ascertainment - Hospital-Discharge-Only

Brief description

Restricted data sets like cancer patients recruited into studies or comprehensive case registries like patient data stored in administrative systems can be used to assess completeness of case registration. It is a precondition that these data sets are not part of the routine registration process; otherwise completeness estimates would be useless. Furthermore it must be assumed that these data sets are nearly 100% complete.

Applicability to the Austrian National Cancer Registry

Applicability is at least partly given as independent data sets are available. Data sets restricted to a tumor site and/or a hospital are sometimes provided by study groups and could be used for completeness estimation, provided that enough information on patient identification is given. However, when using these data sets it is not possible to estimate or compare completeness on Austrian wide level. Hospital discharge data are available for all hospitals in Austria but information on patient identification is restricted. As soon as a routine for record-linkage of Austrian hospital discharge data with Austrian National Cancer Registry data is available, a Hospital-Discharge-Only (HDO) index can be calculated to assess completeness.

Suitability for routine use

The challenge after establishing a method for record-linkage is its realization. Dealing with huge data sets (more than 2.5m hospital discharges per year, thereof more than 12% discharges with a cancer diagnose, compiled for many years) an outstanding technical support is needed. If data volume can be managed and the risks caused by record linkage are considered the use of hospital discharge data for completeness control can be implemented into routine.

Reasons for (non-)inclusion into the study

This quantitative method was included into the study because it provides numerical estimates for completeness. Furthermore, the method does not rely on assumptions that are to be accepted blindly. The only assumption – record-linkage – can be kept under control through appropriate assumptions. From using hospital discharge data as independent data set, clear statements concerning the completeness on national and regional level can be expected.

2.2.10 Capture–recapture methods

Brief description

Capture-recapture methods, primarily used for wildlife population censuses, have also been used for the estimation of completeness of case ascertainment of cancer registries. Two or more independent sources providing incomplete lists of cancer patients are linked. E.g., with two sources four combinations are possible: the patient is listed in both data sets (a), only in the first (b), only in the second (c) or in none of them (d). The number of all patients (a+b+c+d) can be estimated by matrix calculation using ((a+b)*(a+c))/a. "Independent sources" means that the identification of a case by one source is independent of the other.

Applicability to the Austrian National Cancer Registry

The Austrian National Cancer Registry cannot easily collect data sets from independent sources on its own. Most independent sources notifying routinely cancer cases to the cancer registry do not cover identical populations. As valid calculation requires that at least some patients are listed in both data sets, the method is not applicable using routine data sets because this requirement is rather unlikely to be met.

Sometimes data sets are provided by study groups. It has to be discussed whether these sets, mostly restricted to a tumor site and/or a hospital, are a good basis for capture-recapture studies. They could be used as one source and the cancer registry as the other. Assuming 100% completeness for these files, the method of independent data sets (as described above) could be applied. To decide which method fits better, further investigation on the files available is needed.

Suitability for routine use

The biggest challenge for routine use is the collection of the data sets as it has to be assumed that all data sets are independent and that all individuals have the same probability of being captured. Both assumptions cannot be directly tested and violations of each could lead to over- or under-estimation of the true patient population size.

Reasons for (non-)inclusion into the study

This method was not included into the study for reasons of applicability and suitability as described above. Nevertheless, it would be very interesting to examine data sets provided by study groups and compare results of independent data sets method with results of capture-recapture method or with other qualified methods.

2.2.11 Death certificate methods - DCN/M:I method

Brief description

Death certificates are sources for cancer registries. They are used as complementary source of information on new cancer cases, for completeness and validity control and for outcome analyses of registered patients. Death-certificate-only cases (DCO) are defined as cases that come to the attention of the cancer registry only by death certificate. Besides DCO the concepts of DCI and DCN exist (death certificate initiated and death certificate notified, respectively).

In order to estimate missing cases, it has to be assumed that case fatality is the same for registered and for unregistered cases. Using matrix calculation on the proportions of unregistered to registered cases before and after DCI trace back the number of missing cases can be estimated. Ajiki et al. (1998) provide a formula for estimating completeness from DCI and the M:I ratio: (1 - DCI * (1/M:I))/(1-DCI), the formula provided in the original publication by Parkin et al. (1994) is wrong (Parkin & Bray, 2009).

Applicability to the Austrian National Cancer Registry

Because of the way cases notified by a regional cancer registry are processed, it is not possible for the Austrian National Cancer Registry to identify DCI or DCN cases for all regions.

Suitability for routine use

If the number of DCI or DCN cases was available, it would be easy to calculate this estimator of completeness. The question is how strong incomplete incidence numbers used in the formula (M:I) bias the estimator.

Schmidtmann (2009) compared various methods for completeness estimation using a simulated cancer registry with known completeness in various registration scenarios. Many methods – thereof three methods related to DCN cases – were included in the analysis. These were (1) DCN-method using the Lincoln-Petersen estimator, (2) DCN-method using the Parkin formula and (3) DCN-method using the modified Parkin formula. The simulated completeness was best estimated by the DCN-method using the modified Parkin formula and two other non DCN-methods. In general, most methods underestimated the true (simulated) completeness, the Lincoln-Petersen estimator even drastically.

Reasons for (non-)inclusion into the study

This method was not included into the study for reasons of applicability as described above.

Furthermore, the definition and interpretation of DCI and DCN cases (death certificate initiated and death certificate notified, respectively) still cause confusion and are used differently in cancer registries. This confusing situation is also found in international literature. Whereas Parkin et al. (1994) refer to DCN cases for the death certificate method, Parkin and Bray (2009) describe the method as follows: "The DC and M:I method requires that death certificate initiated (DCI) cases can be explicitly identified by the registry, and makes use of the mortality: incidence ratio (M:I) to estimate the proportion of the initially unregistered cancer cases that do not die."

2.2.12 Death certificate methods - The Flow Method

Brief description

The Flow Method is based on the logical flow of data in the registration system and on the time distribution of various probabilities inherent in this flow. To estimate completeness of cancer registry data, the number of patients not registered after a given period of time after diagnosis of cancer has to be ascertained. These patients are divided into two groups: patients that are alive and still unregistered (missing) and patients who died without being registered during life and remained unregistered because cancer was not mentioned on the death certificate (lost). This method does not require that DCI cases are explicitly enumerated and it is not sensitive to the proportion of DCIs or to the assumption of equal M:I ratios in cases that are, or are not, traced.

Applicability to the Austrian National Cancer Registry

The Flow Method is currently of limited suitability because of two basic assumptions. First, the date of registration is an important parameter within the Flow Method. It is used for calculating the time distributions required for completeness estimation. However, owing to the Austrian cancer data transfer procedures, only the registration date in the Austrian National Cancer Registry – but not the primarily registration date in the regional registries – is available. This effect of delay could be partly settled using proxies. The second important parameter, survival time, is most likely biased by incompleteness.

Suitability for routine use

The Flow Method relies only on routinely registered data and can therefore be executed rapidly and inexpensively. If an appropriate registration date and valid estimators of survival were available, it would be easy to apply. Another advantage is that it is a quantitative method, providing a numerical estimator of completeness.

Reasons for (non-)inclusion into the study

Despite the reasons mentioned in "applicability", the method was used in the study as it seems worth testing the suitability of the Flow Method for the Austrian National Cancer Registry in the sense of a method study. Results have to be interpreted carefully.

2.3 Definitions

2.3.1 Tumor entities

For analysis ICD-10 codes were grouped according to table 2.

Table 2: ICD-10 codes and texts used for grouping tumor sites for analysis (ICD-10, 1998)

ICD-10 code	ICD-10 text
C00-C97 except C44	Malignant neoplasms (excluding non-melanoma skin cancer)
C00-C14	Malignant neoplasms of lip, oral cavity and pharynx
C15-C26	Malignant neoplasms of digestive organs
C30-C39	Malignant neoplasms of respiratory and intrathoracic organs
C40-C41	Malignant neoplasms of bone and articular cartilage
C43	Melanoma of skin
C45-C49	Malignant neoplasms of mesothelial and soft tissue
C50	Malignant neoplasm of breast
C51-C58	Malignant neoplasms of female genital organs
C60-C63	Malignant neoplasms of male genital organs
C64-C68	Malignant neoplasms of urinary tract
C69-C72	Malignant neoplasms of eye, brain and other parts of central nervous system
C73-C75	Malignant neoplasms of thyroid and other endocrine glands

2.3.2 Age-adjustment

To allow for international comparison the world standard population (Segi, 1960) was used for age-adjustment (table 3). Age-adjustment for sex specific tumor sites as "female breast", "female genital organs" and "male genital organs" refers to the corresponding population of women and men, respectively.

Table 3: World standard population (Segi, 1960) and annual average Austrian population 2008 (Statistik Austria, 2013)

Age group	SEGI world standard population	Annual average population Austria 2008
0 to 4 years	12,000	396,483
5 to 9 years	10,000	409,752
10 to 14 years	9,000	463,321
15 to 19 years	9,000	501,117
20 to 24 years	8,000	519,599
25 to 29 years	8,000	545,638
30 to 34 years	6,000	539,134
35 to 39 years	6,000	640,746
40 to 44 years	6,000	715,334
45 to 49 years	6,000	671,507
50 to 54 years	5,000	561,512
55 to 59 years	4,000	491,924
60 to 64 years	4,000	442,598
65 to 69 years	3,000	476,434
70 to 74 years	2,000	299,211
75 to 79 years	1,000	276,178
80 to 84 years	500	217,964
85 and over	500	168,097

2.3.3 Test of significance

No tests of significance as described in Cancer Incidence in Five Continents (Parkin, Whelan, Ferlay, Teppo and Thomas, 2002) were conducted because the grouping by region, gender and tumor site would have caused too many significance tests. Alpha accumulation would lead to many significant results by chance or result in very low levels of significance. Furthermore, different population sizes of the federal states are problematic for tests of significance. To establish a basic overview of the completeness of available cancer data time trends were used as starting points. Whenever possible, confidence intervals were calculated.

3 Results by findings

3.1 Time series

Many of plausible de- or increases of cancer incidence rates which are not related to completeness alterations were found. However, some time periods showed changes of incidence rates most likely related to changes of completeness.

Fluctuations of cancer incidence rates and regional variability in the first ten years of the available data (1983-1993) were shown. These were explained by an increase in completeness of case ascertainment due to quality improvement during the early development stage of the Austrian National Cancer Registry and the four regional cancer registries. Figure 4 exemplifies this, showing cancer incidence rates and M:I ratios for Austria and for Tyrol for the years 1983 to 1992. Whereas cancer incidence rates and M:I ratios changed suddenly, survival time (five year cumulative relative survival) increased slowly.

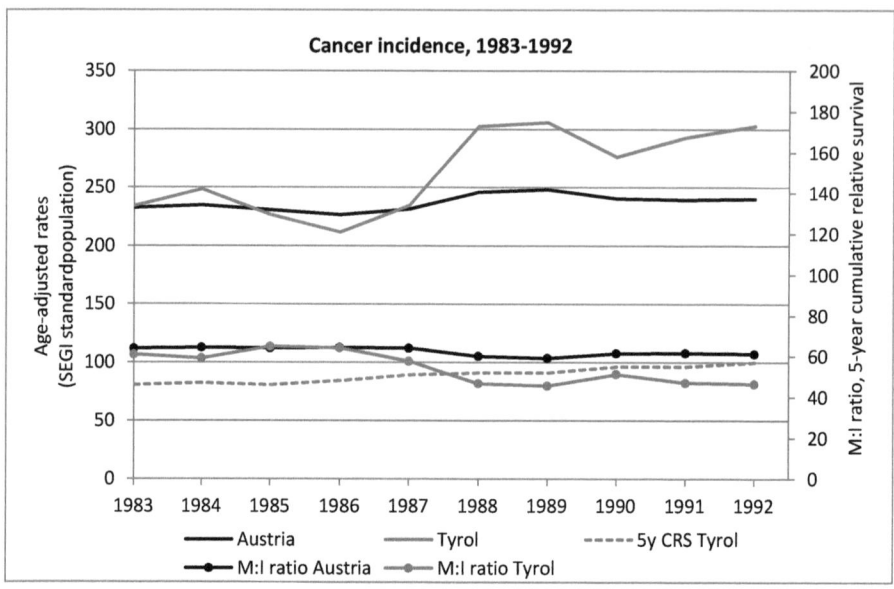

Figure 4: Cancer incidence, M:I ratio, 5-year cumulative relative survival, Austria and Tyrol, 1983-1992 (per 24.09.2012)

From 1991 to 1997 cancer incidence increased steadily. The reason for the increase could not be allocated definitely. An increase of cancer incidence seems as plausible as an increase in completeness of case ascertainment. HDO indices showed random variation which is a sign for stable completeness. M:I ratio was not conducive to interpretation as the long-term decrease of M:I ratio could be explained by increasing completeness or increasing survival time observed during these years. However, the increase in cancer incidence in 1993 and 1997 is primarily caused by a regional increase of completeness of case ascertainment in Carinthia (1993) and in Vienna (1997). Non-recurring efforts to increase data quality and data completeness in both federal states caused incidence peaks in the years mentioned. Figure 5 shows age adjusted cancer incidence rates, M:I ratios and HDO indices for Austria, Carinthia and Vienna.

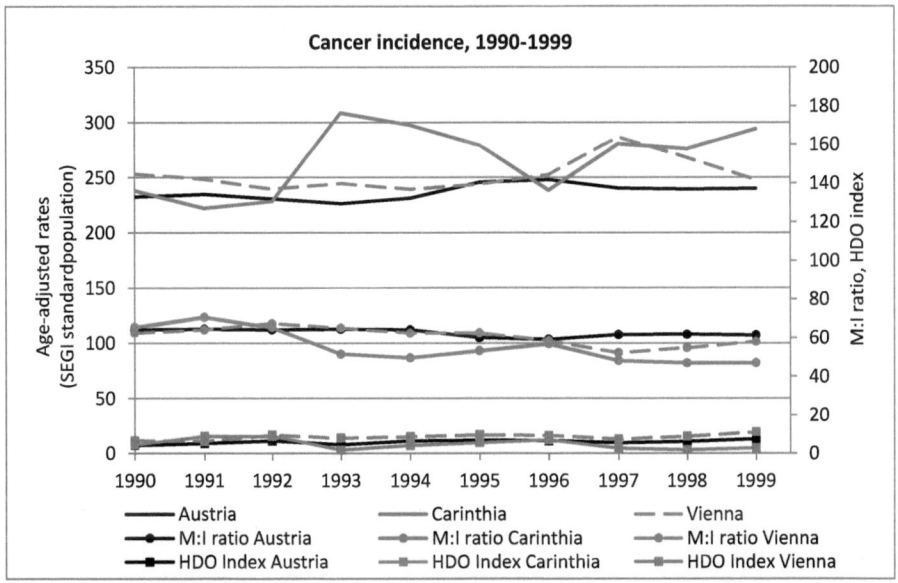

Figure 5: Cancer incidence, M:I ratio, HDO index, Austria, Carinthia and Vienna, 1990-1999 (per 24.09.2012)

From 1997 until 2004, cancer incidence rates were rather stable with the exception of Vorarlberg. The peak there was caused by an increase in prostate cancer due to screening. Do stable rates reflect stable conditions of cancer risk or increasing cancer risk masked by decreasing completeness? HDO indices increased slightly arguing for a little decrease of completeness. M:I ratio decreased even less slightly. A slight decrease could result from increasing completeness or from increasing survival times. Most likely this small alteration can be explained by decreasing completeness overlapped by increasing survival time.

Since 2005 cancer incidence rates have been decreasing and M:I ratios have been rather stable but the HDO indices have been increasing. The decrease of cancer incidence rates in the last published years can be partly explained with a long-standing reduction of cancer cases for several sites (Figure 6) and partly with regional incompleteness. The long-standing reduction of gastric cancer, cancer of the cervix and cancer of the ovary is not visible in the total number of cancer. It is compensated by a massive increase in prostate cancer. The reduction of prostate cancer since 2004 reduces the total number of cancer cases as well. This seems to be a result of more frequent screening rather than a sign for incompleteness.

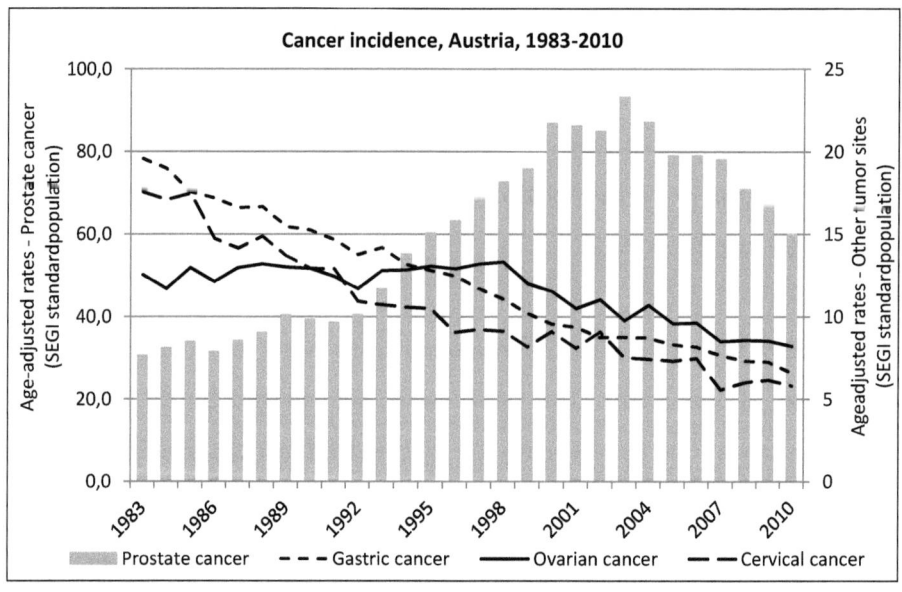

Figure 6: Incidence of gastric cancer, cancer of the cervix and the ovary and prostate cancer, Austria, 1983-2010 (per 24.09.2012)

The decrease of cancer incidence rates in the last two published years is most likely a result of incompleteness as M:I ratio and HDO indices increase suddenly. The Flow Method as well as the comparison of the yearly snapshots of the cancer registry's database show the lack of completeness of case ascertainment in the most recent years in a very impressive way (Figure 7).

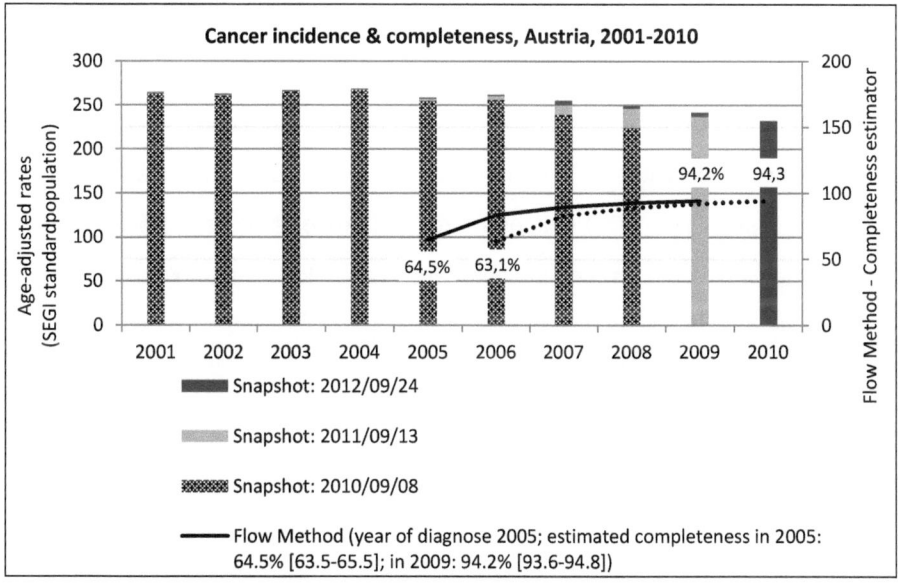

Figure 7: Cancer incidence 2001-2010 (per 08.09.2010, 13.09.2011 and 24.09.2012 respectively) and completeness estimator using the Flow Method (years of diagnose 2005 and 2006), Austria

3.2 Regional pattern

Usually, differences in incidence rates result from differences in completeness. Most indices used for estimation of completeness confirm the assumption that higher incidence rates result from higher completeness and vice versa. Federal states results´ are shown only for all tumor sites combined.

The federal state with the most complete cancer incidence data was **Tyrol**. Constantly highest incidence rates since 1988 were reflected in constantly lowest M:I ratios as well as lowest HDO indices. Results of the Flow Method were not valid due to violation of assumptions. The very high completeness of case ascertainment already shown by the Tyrolean Cancer Registry (Oberaigner, 2009) was verified. **Carinthia** also has very complete cancer incidence data. The year 1993 shows a peak. From 2000 on, a period of high completeness of case ascertainment is shown. Looking at age-adjusted cancer incidence rates, M:I ratios and HDO indices a very clear picture is seen. M:I ratios and HDO indices mirror incidence rates on a horizontal axis, thus showing that these indices are valid to estimate completeness (Figure 8).

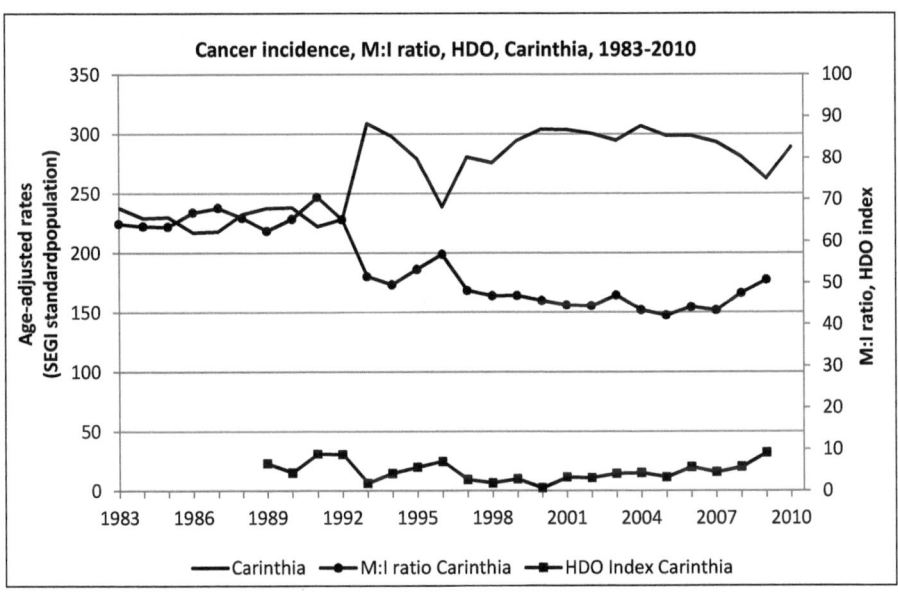

Figure 8: Cancer incidence, M:I ratio, HDO index, Carinthia, 1983-2010 (per 24.09.2012)

A similar pattern showing high completeness of case ascertainment since 2001 was seen in **Vorarlberg**. The increase of incidence rates seen in the years following 2001 did not reflect an increase of completeness but increasing incidence rates of prostate cancer. Therefore the later decrease of incidence rates was not a completeness problem but a typical pattern related to screening. Nevertheless, completeness in the most recent year of diagnosis is limited because regional cancer registries complete data only after publishing by the Austrian National Cancer Registry. In the following year's snapshot published by the Austrian National Cancer Registry these data are available. Temporarily, regional incompleteness and efforts on regional level to increase completeness are shown for Carinthia, Vorarlberg, and Styria (Figure 9).

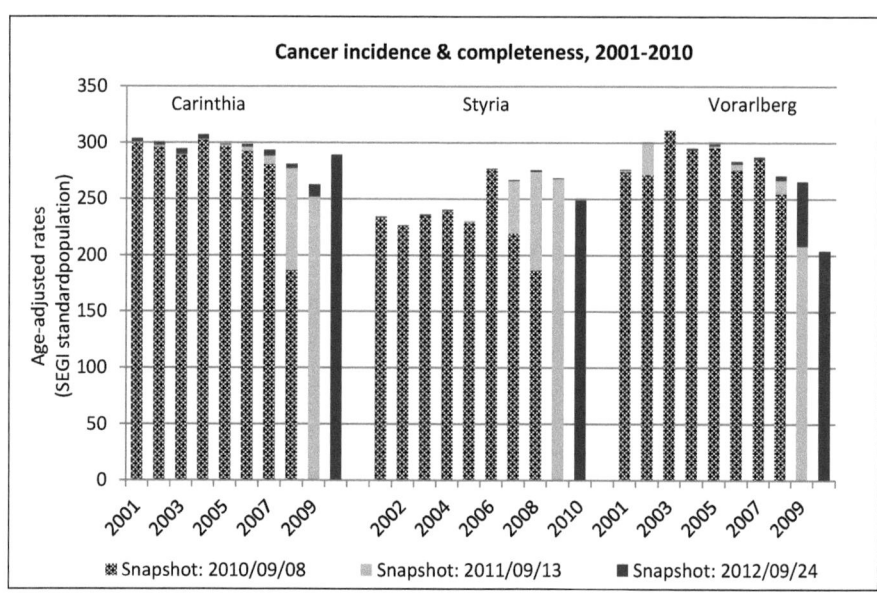

Figure 9: Cancer incidence 2001-2010 (per 08.09.2010, 13.09.2011 and 24.09.2012 respectively), Carinthia, Styria, and Vorarlberg

All **Salzburg** indices show a satisfactory completeness of case ascertainment between 1999 and 2004. In the following years completeness slowly decreased and since 2007 an obvious decrease of completeness of case ascertainment has been seen in Salzburg – a federal state that collects cancer incidence data in a regional registry such as Tyrol, Carinthia and Vorarlberg (Figure 10). Similar patterns of age-adjusted incidence rates, M:I ratios and HDO indices were seen in **Burgenland**, **Lower Austria** and **Upper Austria**. All these federal states do not collect cancer incidence data via a regional cancer registry. It is remarkable that in Burgenland the absolute number of HDO cases is not large enough to settle the deficiency estimated by keeping M:I ratio constant for the most recent years. An explanation for this result is that patients are diagnosed and treated in other federal states but not notified by those.

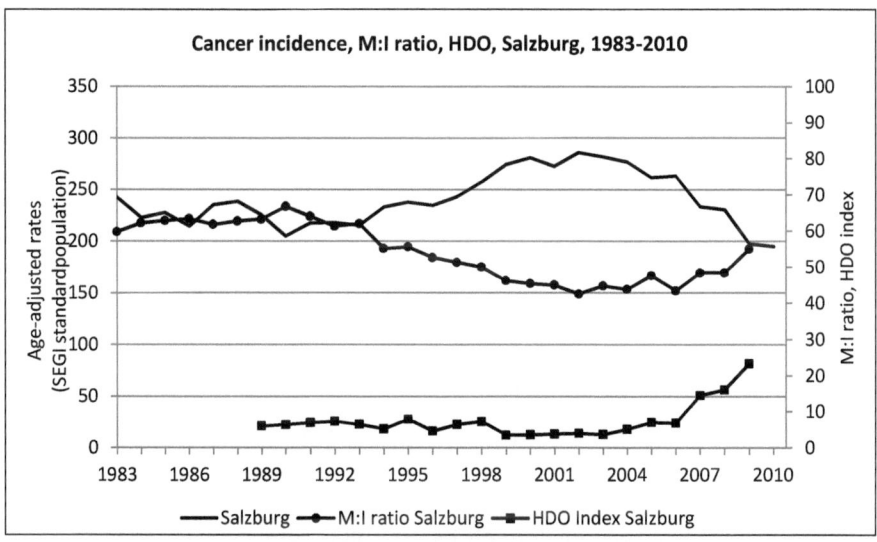

Figure 10: Cancer incidence, M:I ratio, HDO index, Salzburg, 1983-2010 (per 24.09.2012)

In contrast to the decrease in completeness in Salzburg, Burgenland, Lower Austria and Upper Austria, completeness of case ascertainment in **Styria** increased in the more recent years. Two departments of pathology were added to the list of departments for routine data collection and the increase in cancer incidence rates was reflected in decreasing M:I ratios as well as in decreasing HDO indices. The increase in cancer incidence rates from 2005 to 2006 and temporary regional incompleteness are shown in Figure 9.

Compared to the other federal states, **Vienna** shows lowest age-adjusted incidence rates and highest M:I ratios and HDO indices. This hints at a rather high incompleteness. However, M:I ratios could be elevated not only by incompleteness but also by high mortality rates and low survival. Probably the results show a combination of low completeness and low survival probabilities in Vienna.

3.3 Tumor sites

The comparison of the incidence rates by tumor sites gives no hints on completeness because the risk for different tumor sites differs clearly. Nevertheless, the comparison of incidence rates of a selected tumor site on a timeline or across regions provides information on completeness. For most of the tumor sites alterations with time are creeping, giving no dedicated hint on a sudden de- or increase of completeness. Furthermore, numbers of incident cases are often very small, thus leading to large confidence intervals. The results of cross regional comparisons of incidence rates are hard to interpret as the rates are not only influenced by completeness of case ascertainment but also by regional cancer risk. For single tumor sites the risk certainly shows more regional variation than for all tumor sites combined. M:I ratio and Flow Method both depend on survival times and thus show the same uncertainties on regional level as described above for cancer risk. HDO index seems to be the only sound method for assessing the completeness on tumor site level. It is not yet sufficiently developed to be used on tumor site level.

The challenge of assessing the completeness of case ascertainment by tumor sites is illustrated by two examples: Female breast cancer in Vienna and lung cancer in Vienna. It is already known that cancer registration in Vienna lacks completeness (Hackl, Klimont, Waldhör, 2011 and Hackl, Zielonke, Waldhör, 2012). Nevertheless, there seem to be differences on the level of completeness of case ascertainment by tumor site.

Completeness of case ascertainment for female breast cancer in Vienna

Since 1990 the age-adjusted incidence rate for female breast cancer in Vienna has been hovering around the Austrian mean whereas the age-adjusted mortality rate is clearly elevated. The application of the Austrian M:I ratio to the Viennese mortality data results in an incidence rate for Vienna which is significantly higher than the cancer registries data (Figure 11). The Flow Method estimates a completeness of 89.9 percent (95% confidence interval: 84.1; 94.6) for female breast cancer in Vienna compared to 92.7 percent for female breast cancer in Austria (95% confidence interval: 88.7; 95.9). Lower completeness in Vienna is seen, although confidence intervals overlap widely.

Basically, two explanations are possible: First, data are complete and survival time of women with breast cancer living in Vienna is significantly lower than survival time of women living in other federal states. Second, survival time in Vienna is the same as in other federal states but many breast cancer cases in women diagnosed or treated in Vienna were not notified to the Austrian National Cancer Registry. The latter explanation seems more plausible, especially with regard to the higher rates in the first years of cancer documentation. However, most likely both explanations contribute to the before-mentioned result.

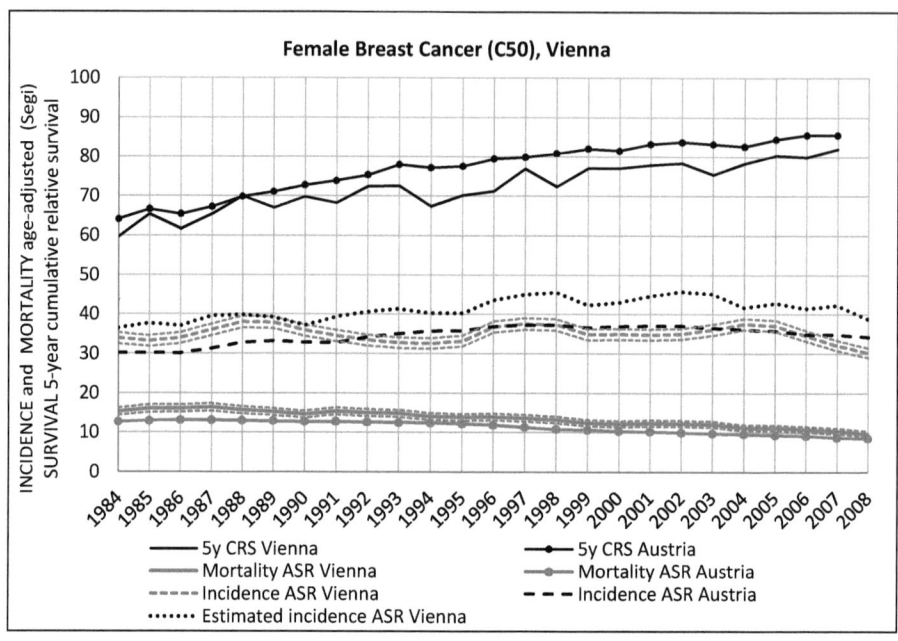

Figure 11: Female breast cancer, cancer incidence, mortality and survival, Austria and Vienna, estimated cancer incidence rate Vienna applying Austrian M:I ratio on Viennese mortality rates, 1984-2008 (per 27.08.2009)

Completeness of case ascertainment for lung cancer in Vienna

Since the Austrian National Cancer Registry published data for the first time, the age-adjusted incidence rate for lung cancer in Vienna has been significantly higher than the Austrian mean. The age-adjusted mortality rate is also clearly elevated. The application of the Austrian M:I ratio to the Viennese mortality data results in an incidence rate for Vienna which is nearly the same as the one of cancer registries data (Figure 12).

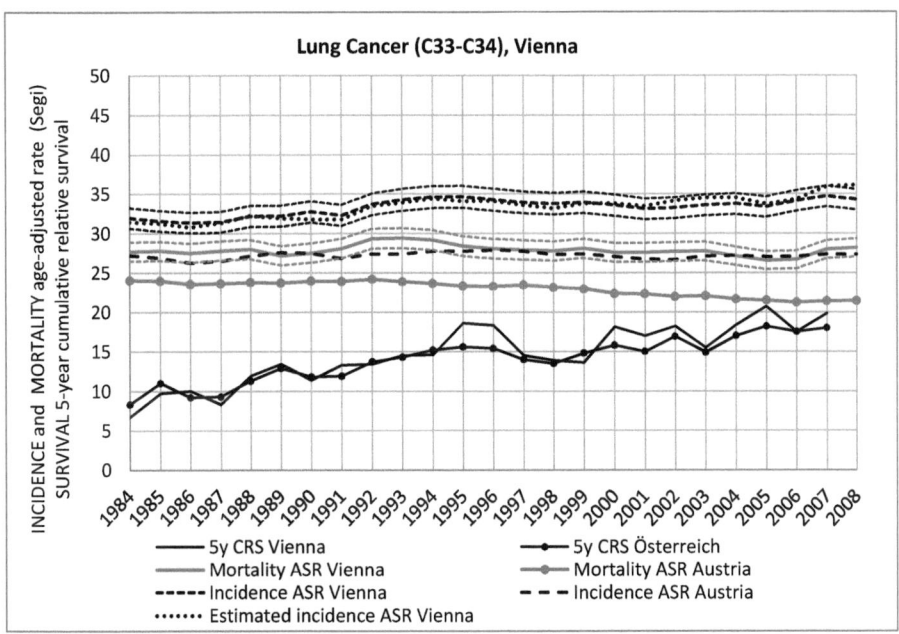

Figure 12: Lung cancer, cancer incidence, mortality and survival, Austria and Vienna, estimated cancer incidence rate Vienna applying Austrian M:I ratio on Viennese mortality rates, 1984-2008 (per 27.08.2009)

The Flow Method estimates a completeness of 96.9 percent (95% confidence interval: 94.4; 98.8) for lung cancer in Vienna compared to 96.8 percent for lung cancer in Austria (95% confidence interval: 95.3; 98.0). M:I ratio and the results of the Flow Method both show high completeness for Viennese lung cancer cases.

Basically, two explanations for this surprising level of completeness are possible: First, low survival of lung cancer patients leads to high completeness because most patients that were not registered during lifetime are notified to the cancer registry via death certificates within a short period of time. This hypothesis is supported by data on pancreas cancer which also show low survival and high completeness of case ascertainment (own calculations, data not shown). Second, lung cancer registration in Vienna benefits from highly committed medical doctors. A Viennese medical study group set up a clinical cancer registry for lung cancer. Although this clinical cancer registry never reached routine status it is likely that awareness for cancer registration is very high within the special field of lung cancer.

4 Discussion

With the exception of the Flow Method´s regional analyses, all completeness estimates show more or less the same level of completeness. Two assumptions could be verified: First, data for federal states showing higher incidence rates are more complete than data for federal states showing lower incidence rates. Second, completeness decreases in the latest published years of diagnoses. It can be assumed that these results are reliable as they are produced using very different concepts for completeness estimation. In addition, analysis showed that the Flow Method was not appropriate for regional completeness estimations of the Austrian National Cancer Registry under current conditions and results are likely to be biased.

4.1 Evaluation of methods

4.1.1 Evaluation of Stability of incidence rates over time, Comparison of incidence rates in different populations

The application of these methods resulted in descriptive analyses of time trends without any numerical estimation of completeness. Nevertheless, these analyses proved to be well suited to establish a basic overview of the available cancer data.

A sudden de- or increase of absolute numbers of cancer cases or incidence rates is most likely a sign of changing completeness. The combination of data analyses and background knowledge of the cancer registry´s history shows that actions to increase completeness resulted in an increase of registered cancer cases. The other way round, irregularities in time trends could mostly be explained by actions increasing completeness or problems resulting in decreasing completeness. Creeping alterations of completeness cannot be identified easily with this method.

A comparison of incidence rates in different populations can indicate varying completeness across regions. For this purpose it has to be assumed that the risk of getting cancer does not differ significantly between the regions compared. On a large perspective this assumption seems plausible if Austria is compared with Western Europe or the federal states within Austria are analyzed. However, this assumption may lead in a wrong direction as one of the main duties of an epidemiological cancer registry is to point out regional differences even for areas believed to have similar risk factors.

4.1.2 Evaluation of Mortality:Incidence ratio

It is obvious to use mortality data in order to assess completeness of incidence data. Nowadays some registries use the M:I ratio to calculate numerical estimators, although Parkin and Bray (2009) consider M:I ratio a qualitative method. I do not recommend to calculate a numerical estimator comparing incidence of selected tumor sites across regions and calculating expected incidence numbers based on the M:I ratio of one region as equal survival rates for all regions under comparison is critical to be assumed. Nevertheless, it could be shown that this method is suited for the completeness evaluation of time series to a certain extent.

Changes of M:I ratio can be explained by changing completeness or changing survival times. The longer patients survive their cancer diagnosis the higher the probability of dying of another cause. Therefore, higher survival rates correlate with lower mortality rates. Assuming constant incidence numbers decreasing mortality leads to a decrease of M:I ratio. The correlation between survival changes and changes of M:I ratio becomes obvious looking at increasing survival in the 1980ies and 1990ies and at the changing pattern of survival of male and female cancer patients. Whereas slow changes of M:I ratio could mask creeping completeness decrease, sudden de- or increases of M:I ratio are most likely a sign of changing completeness.

The comparison of M:I ratios across regions is problematic as no reference values exist and survival probabilities confound the results. Assuming that mortality rates are correct and survival rates do not differ between regions, higher M:I ratios are to be explained by lower incidence rates, i.e. lower completeness of case ascertainment. If equal survival rates cannot be assumed different regional M:I ratios can be explained either by different completeness or by different survival times.

4.1.3 Evaluation of the Flow Method

The Flow Method turns out to be a very interesting method for completeness estimation by cancer registries, providing a numerical estimator of completeness. Relying only on routinely registered data it can be executed rapidly and inexpensively in routine data analysis.

This method divides an ideal 100 percent complete database into three fractions: The first fraction, registered cases, represents completeness of case ascertainment. The second fraction, missing cases, consists of cancer cases still alive but not registered in the cancer registry. The third fraction, lost cases, covers patients who have died without being registered during life and remain unregistered because cancer was not mentioned on the death certificate. The Flow Method estimates the probabilities for missing and lost cases for many points in time, calculates a completeness estimator and depicts it on a time line. Calculation is done by subtracting one minus the probability for missing and minus the probability for lost cases. A confidence interval for the completeness estimator can be calculated as well.

Whereas the idea is rather simple, the model is complex and based on assumptions not easy to test. Assumptions which cannot be met bias the results to an unknown extent. Obviously invalid assumptions for the Austrian database were investigated in the present study, but still more work is needed to gain a valid estimator of completeness. The inclusion of survival time calculated from the registry's data seems problematic for regions or tumor sites with systematic incompleteness. If for example long time survivors are missing in the registry, survival time is underestimated. According to the assumptions incorporated into the Flow Method, lower survival time leads to higher completeness estimates. Applying the Flow Method on tumor level this bias does not attract attention as it amplifies the expected results. Analysis of Austrian cancer data on regional level showed that regions with assumedly higher completeness of case ascertainment seem to have higher survival rates and the Flow Method's completeness estimator was lower than for regions with assumedly lower completeness.

4.1.4 Evaluation of the concept of Hospital-Discharge-Only (HDO)

The approach of completeness estimation using hospital discharge data seems very promising and should be pursued after evaluation of record linkage. It shall be based on a non-controversial record linkage by a unique identifier as soon as possible. As the Flow Method, the Hospital-Discharge-Only index provides a numerical estimator of completeness. Since it relies on already available electronic data only it can be executed rapidly and inexpensively in routine data analysis.

The Hospital-Discharge-Only index (HDO index) mimics the idea of the death-certificate-only index (DCO index). The DCO index – the percentage of DCO cases to total registrations (including DCO cases) - is well known as quality indicator for cancer registries. It shows the proportion of cases not registered while the patients were living. The HDO index is defined as the percentage of Hospital-Discharge-Only cases to the total number of cancer cases available. Total registrations include all cases that should be published as cancer incidence statistics, i.e. registered-in-life cases (RIL cases), death-certificate-notified cases (DCN cases), DCO cases and HDO cases.

Although the present numerical estimators definitely underestimate completeness, they show the same patterns as other methods (Hackl, Klimont, Waldhör, 2011 and Hackl, Zielonke, Waldhör, 2012). However, record linkage described in the presented work needs further investigation.

4.2 Further Perspectives

4.2.1 Retain already established analyses and strengthen standardized routine jobs

I recommend continuing the use of "Stability of incidence rates over time" and "Comparison of incidence rates in different populations" for completeness assessment. These methods are already applied in the Austrian National Cancer Registry, but require a much higher degree of standardization and automation. Descriptive time series analyses should be based on routinely prepared standardized charts causing little effort and being unchanged from one year to another. These charts shall be prepared for all malignant tumors combined, for selected tumor sites and for all malignant tumors combined excluding selected tumor sites (e.g. prostate cancer) and broken down by sex and by federal state respectively. Charts should include incidence and mortality rates and related indicators as survival and prevalence as well as the Mortality:Incidence ratio and the percentage of DCO cases. Furthermore, incidence rates for one published year of diagnosis in various consecutive snap shots of the cancer registry´s data base should be compared routinely to estimate the time span it takes to complete the data for a year of diagnosis.

4.2.2 Investigate the Flow Method

Impact of delayed registration date

The major problem of adopting the Flow Method for the Austrian National Cancer Registry is the item "date of registration of a cancer case in the cancer registry". Its importance for the estimation of the probability of non-registration while surviving – a parameter used to estimate completeness – has already been mentioned in the introduction of the paper "Estimation of completeness of case ascertainment of Austrian cancer incidence data using the Flow Method". Within the Austrian National Cancer Registry only the date of registration in the registry is stored. For the federal states providing cancer data through a regional registry the available registration date shows a delay compared to the original date of registration in the regional registry. For a description of the Austrian registration process and the anticipated effect of the delayed registration date see methods section of the referred paper.

To correct the effect of the delayed registration date, a second calculation was conducted using the same value for the probability of non-registration while surviving for all federal states. The results are presented in the mentioned paper as well. The unexpectedly low completeness estimators for data provided by the regional registries of Tyrol and Vorarlberg increased to comparable values using the same value for the probability of non-registration while surviving for all federal states. Based on previous analyses, not only comparable but even higher completeness has been expected for Tyrol and Vorarlberg.

Impact of survival time

The second important parameter used for completeness estimation is survival time. I assume that high survival leads to more missing cases as long term survivors are not reported via death certificates within a reasonable time span. As survival times in Tyrol and Vorarlberg are much higher than e.g. in Vienna, Lower Austria and Styria (5-year cumulative relative survival, 2002-2006, all sites together), completeness could either be underestimated for Tyrol and Vorarlberg or overestimated for the other federal states.

Work in progress / further tasks

Both limitations of the study (delayed registration date and impact of survival time) were discussed in the mentioned paper. Further investigation on the registration date is still to be done. The influences of survival time on the completeness estimator as well as the influence of completeness of case ascertainment on the calculated survival times have to be tested in detail.

After discussion of the before mentioned paper with representatives of the regional registries, it was agreed that the problem of delayed registration date should be solved sustainably as the Flow Method is still a very promising tool for completeness evaluation. As a first step the regional registries will check their database for the registration date. If available, they will provide rules about how the date is defined and the date itself to be added to the Austrian National Cancer Registry in retrospect. Afterwards, the Flow Method will be conducted again using the adopted data set and the results will be discussed with the regional registries before publication. In future a harmonized definition of the date of registration shall be developed and the interface for data delivery to the Austrian National Cancer Registry shall be adapted.

Based on the results of the Flow Method applied on the adapted data set the impact of survival differences needs to be assessed. As described elsewhere (Statistik Austria, 2012), it is assumed that survival differences between the federal states can partly be explained by incompleteness of data. The use of survival time for completeness estimations within the Flow Method results in a vicious circle. Therefore, it is necessary to investigate on regional survival estimation. A workshop on survival estimation will be held by the Austrian National Cancer Registry and the regional cancer registries. Regional differences in survival times could result from differences in healthcare, therapy, screening (i.e. lead time bias and length time bias) and overdiagnosis, or be caused artificially by different levels of completeness of case ascertainment. The workshop's results are to be incorporated in the interpretation of the Flow Method's results.

4.2.3 Enhance the concept of Hospital-Discharge-Only (HDO)

Impact of missing unique identifiers

The major problem using hospital discharge data for completeness estimation is the lack of unique identifiers. Neither can discharge cases belonging to the same person be condensed into one discharge data set nor is any reliable identifier available to link the data to the cancer registry. The challenge of condensing and linking the data set is to set up rules that are strong enough to avoid wrong record linkage (resulting in completeness overestimation) but also soft enough not to miss too much true combinations (resulting in completeness underestimation). This has already been discussed in paper "Austrian cancer data completeness, referring to hospital discharge data - The challenge of record linkage"

Work in progress / further tasks

The before-mentioned paper leads to five topics that will be investigated by the Austrian National Cancer Registry step by step within the near future. The key items are testing and improving the record linkage and thereby assessing the quality and usability of the hospital discharge data for this task. Furthermore, hospital discharge data will be used to identify systematic patterns of incompleteness. This knowledge enables the Austrian National Cancer Registry to increase the reporting discipline constituted by national law. Information gained by the concept of HDO will be used to extrapolate incidence numbers to settle the assessed incompleteness in the latest published years of diagnoses as well as completeness differences across federal states as far as possible. The impact of the estimated incompleteness on survival time calculations will be assessed. Last but not least Hospital-Discharge-Only cases could be used to gain further information on the missed cancer cases from hospitals. This would directly improve completeness and data quality of the Austrian National Cancer Registry.

Testing and improving record linkage, quality and usability of hospital discharge data

The analysis of the record linkage between hospital data and cancer registry data showed that not only hospital data but also cancer registry cases failed linkage. Unlinked hospital discharge data potentially identify cases missing in the cancer registry. For unlinked cancer registry cases it is assumed that record linkage rules were too rigid. As a result, cancer cases (usually only notified via hospitals) could not be linked to the corresponding discharge file.

Currently, in an ongoing project, samples of unlinked hospital discharge data sets are checked in various hospitals across Austria. The information gained through this work will help to improve the algorithm underlying record linkage and to assess the quality and usability of the hospital discharge data for this method. Adopting the algorithm will bring the hospital discharge index to a more valid numeric estimator of completeness, being a sound fundament for further work as well.

Identify systematic patterns of incompleteness and increasing the reporting discipline

The analysis of the assumed deficiency will possibly show systematic patterns of non-reporting which can be used to improve reporting discipline. Systematic reasons underlying incompleteness could be missing cancer notifications for certain tumor entities or for certain patient groups. It is likely that certain patient groups such as very old cancer patients or patients with a very bad or a very good prognosis are reported more seldom to the registry. This knowledge can lead to strategic actions which increase completeness and quality of the Austrian National Cancer Registry.

Extrapolate incidence numbers to settle the assessed incompleteness

Assuming that the algorithm underlying record linkage is sufficiently valid and the quality and usability of the hospital discharge data for this task is evaluated, the assumed deficiency will be used to estimate the true incidence based on cancer registry data and Hospital-Discharge-Only data.

Assess the impact of the estimated incompleteness on calculated survival time

Comparing survival time across federal states, clearly different survival rates are seen. Basically, access to health care including cancer diagnosis and cancer therapy should largely be the same in all federal states. Therefore, similar survival times for all federal states are expected. The hypothesis that incompleteness biases survival calculation could be tested by calculating survival rates for the estimated incidence based on the enlarged database using Hospital-Discharge-Only data and causes of death statistics.

Improve completeness and data quality of the Austrian National Cancer Registry directly via data recall

Corresponding to the concept of Death-Certificate-Only also Hospital-Discharge-Only cases could be traced back. A death-certificate-only case is a cancer case which came to the attention of the cancer registry only because of cancer being mentioned on the death certificate. The information gained from the death certificate is sent to the hospital which notified the death requesting it to provide more information on the cancer case as for example date of diagnosis or histology. Once the record linkage is validated the same procedure can be established for the Hospital-Discharge-Only cases.

4.3 Strengths and limitations of this study

Completeness of case ascertainment of cancer registry data is difficult to assess and even more difficult to quantify. Various methods for completeness estimation were published, using qualitative and quantitative approaches. Nevertheless, all methods lead to results that can only serve as approximations.

Qualitative estimation-methods are a basis for data exploration. The application of these methods helps to receive an impression of data completeness. However, it seems problematic that these methods are based on assumptions that cannot be tested easily. Although assumptions like a stable time trend or negligible regional differences are reasonable, these assumptions could lead to statistics based more on expectations than reflecting true trends or differences.

Quantitative estimation-methods produce numeric results with positions after the decimal point that might feign higher correctness. These methods rely even more on assumptions than qualitative estimation-methods. In addition, these assumptions are more complex as the assumptions mentioned above. Furthermore, quantitative estimation-methods face some restrictions inherited in the available data.

The present study is an important basis for the Austrian National Cancer Registry's quality management. While many checks for consistency and plausibility were implemented in the cancers registry's software, completeness of case ascertainment was never investigated systematically. However, estimation of completeness of case ascertainment is very important for cancer registries as meaningful regional comparisons of cancer incidence and all further analysis (e.g., comparison of survival rates) are only possible if the completeness of case ascertainment is known.

The study was conducted in the close surrounding of the Austrian National Cancer Registry. This has the advantage that data usually not available for the public could be used, allowing more complex analysis. The allocation of the study at the Medical University of Vienna guarantees objectivity.

The objectives of the study were met. For the first time various science-based methods for completeness estimation were systematically applied on Austrian National Cancer Registry's data. The present study is a quotable assessment of the completeness of case ascertainment of the Austrian National Cancer Registry, describing completeness variations in time, between regions or between tumor sites.

"The study's findings shall be used to develop a meaningful instrument for completeness estimation out of the repertoire of applicable methods to enable further investigation to estimate precise and valid figures for the completeness of case ascertainment on a national level and for each federal state and to extrapolate cancer incidence data equivalent to a 100% complete data base" [see Objectives]. The study's findings can be, and are already, used as a basis for a standard quality report and as described in the chapters "Work in progress / further tasks" for the Flow Method and the concept of Hospital-Discharge-Only (HDO).

5 Conclusion

The decrease of completeness since year of diagnosis 2005 partly results from plausible decrease of cancer incidence for various tumor sites and partly is due to a creeping completeness decrease. Completeness of the two most recently published years is lower than completeness for the years published before. This is shown in all descriptive analyses and becomes particularly obvious when using the Flow Method. Consecutive yearly snapshots of the database show that completeness for a selected year of diagnosis increases with time. The very short time lag between year of diagnosis and year of publication (1 year and 8 months) is the main reason for this result.

Regionally higher cancer incidence rates for all tumors combined result from higher completeness in the regions concerned. Higher cancer incidence rates for all tumors combined frequently are associated with existence of a regional cancer registry. However, data from regional cancer registries sometimes are subject to a longer time lag, contributing to lower overall completeness in the last two published years. The benefits of a regional cancer registry such as smaller population covered and geographical proximity can be transferred to better data quality only if they are combined with outstanding personal commitment. If people in the clinical setting were convinced of the meaningfulness of cancer registration and of the importance of their input and a reasonable allocation of staff to set up an adequate infrastructure was available, data of equal quality could be gained without regional cancer registries.

Completeness estimates for selected cancer sites show expected results. Completeness tends to be higher for cancer sites with lower survival and vice versa.

Valid numerical estimators of completeness are necessary for extrapolation to achieve regionally comparable cancer incidence data and related indicators. However, numerical completeness estimators generated in the study are not valid. Their quality depends on the method used. In order to establish valid estimators investigations into the Flow Method and the concept of Hospital-Discharge-Only are necessary.

Which method(s) should be used in future? This question cannot be answered by a simple recommendation of one or two methods. Various methods are based on assumptions that cannot be tested easily and their validity may vary across cancer registries, depending e.g. on registration methods. The assumption of equal risk factors or equal survival probabilities increases uncertainty. Completeness estimation for time series seems to be easier than regional comparisons as the factor "region" adds confounders like varying risk factors or varying oncological care, resulting in different survival probabilities. These confounders may also change by time but alterations are more evident. However, interpretation of descriptive or numerical completeness estimations needs broad background knowledge on screening activity, on registration processes and on actions taken to increase data quality and completeness.

To quickly discover decreasing completeness, stability of incidence rates over time seems appropriate. This method can be applied easily and results can be used for further investigations to increase completeness of case ascertainment systematically. Nevertheless, it cannot be used to assess the overall level of completeness. For extrapolation to 100 per cent complete data sets valid numerical estimators are needed. Extrapolation could be reached by applying the concept of Hospital-Discharge-Only or the Flow Method. Both methods require further investigations. If a suitable record linkage was established for the concept of Hospital-Discharge-Only, this method would allow a characterization of missing cases and their addition to the cancer registry. This procedure is comparable to the handling of Death-Certificate-Only cases. Further data analyses are to be done on the level of single tumor sites.

M:I ratio is promising for analyses of completeness of case ascertainment but in my opinion it is only of limited suitability to estimate dimensions of expected incidence. It is not suited to compare completeness on a regional level. It is not valid to extrapolate mortality data to incidence data assuming equal regional survival and afterwards use the extrapolated data set to look for regional survival differences. Some of the methods not applied in the study could also add information to investigation on regional completeness differences for selected tumor sites. Furthermore, a detailed analysis of multiple primaries is highly recommended. The percentage of multiple primaries varies between regions and hints on varying completeness of case ascertainment.

Tasks subsequent to this study should be processed as outlined in the discussion. Summing up, these are the continuation of already established methods and the strengthening of standardized routine jobs as well as further investigation into the Flow Method and into Hospital-Discharge-Only. It is highly recommended to document the results of time series analyses and of all other further routinely conducted methods in a structured form. For this purpose a standard quality report mainly consisting of tables and figures should be developed. This quality report should be routinely prepared by the Austrian National Cancer Registry once a year. A summary of the main results should be discussed with regional experts in cancer registration and afterwards be published and sent to all institutions obliged to notify cancer cases.

Results and implications of this study are to be discussed with experts in cancer registration and experts in oncology. It is recommended to establish a "Cancer Data Quality Study Group" consisting of members of the Austrian National Cancer Registry and representatives of the Austrian regional cancer registries. This study group should be extended step by step so that finally all federal states are represented. The study group´s first task should be the investigation into the association of completeness and survival: "Are regional survival differences a result of different regional completeness of cancer registration?"

It seems necessary to explain the standard quality report and the findings of the Cancer Data Quality Study Group to as many people as possible to raise awareness of the cancer registry and of the quality of cancer statistics. As a consequence personal commitment from various players is supposed to rise and improve the quality of cancer statistics sustainably.

6 References

Ajiki W., Tsukuma H., Oshima A. (1998). Index for evaluating completeness of registration in population-based cancer registries and estimation of registration rate at the Osaka Cancer Registry between 1966 and 1992 using this index. Nippon Koshu Eisei Zasshi, 45, 1011–7.

Berrino F., De Angelis R., Sant M., Rosso S., Lasota MB., Coebergh JW., et al.. (2007). Survival for eight major cancers and all cancers combined for European adults diagnosed in 1995-99: results of the EUROCARE-4 study. Lancet Oncology, 8, 773-83.

Bauer A., Kytir J. (2010). Sterbefälle auf ausländischem Staatsgebiet; Erweiterung der Datengrundlage der Gestorbenenstatistik. Statistische Nachrichten, 5, 376-382.

Brenner H. (1995). Limitations of the death certificate only index as a measure of incompleteness of cancer registration. British Journal of Cancer, 72, 506–10.

Brenner H., Hakulinen T. (2005). Population-based monitoring of cancer patient survival in situations with imperfect completeness of cancer registration. British Journal of Cancer, 92, 576-579.

Bullard J., Coleman MP., Robinson D., Lutz JM., Bell J., Peto J. (2000). Completeness of cancer registration: a new method for routine use. British Journal of Cancer, 82, 1111–16.

Bundesministerium für Gesundheit, Krebsrahmenprogramm, Ist-Stands Bericht der Onkologie, unveröffentlichtes Arbeitspapier, 2012.

Concord study, http://www.lshtm.ac.uk/eph/ncde/cancersurvival/research/concord/concord_2.html (23.08.2013).

Curado MP., Edwards B., Shin HR., Storm H., Ferlay J., Heanue M., Boyle P. (2007). Cancer Incidence in Five Continents Vol. IX, IARC Scientific Publication No. 160. Lyon: IARC.

Dickman, P., http://www.pauldickman.com/ (23.08.2013).

Ederer F., Axtell LM., Cutler SJ. (1961). The relative survival rate: a statistical methodology. Journal of the National Cancer Institute Monographs, 6, 101-21.

E-Government-Gesetz - Bundesgesetz über Regelungen zur Erleichterung des elektronischen Verkehrs mit öffentlichen Stellen (E-Government-Gesetz - E-GovG) StF: BGBl. I Nr. 10/2004, http://www.ris.bka.gv.at/Dokument.wxe?Abfrage=BgblAuth&Dokumentnummer=BGBLA_2004_I_10 (23.08.2013).

Hackl M., Klimont J., Waldhör T. (2011). Vollzähligkeitsanalyse der Krebsinzidenz, Methode: Stabilität im Zeitverlauf. Statistische Nachrichten, 9, 848–59.

Hackl M., Waldhoer T. (2012). Estimation of completeness of case ascertainment of Austrian cancer incidence data using the flow method. European Journal of Public Health, Epub ahead of print.

Hackl M., Zielonke N., Waldhör T. (2012). Vollzähligkeitsanalyse der österreichischen Krebsinzidenz Methode: Mortality/Incidence-Ratio. Statistische Nachrichten, 8, 568-77.

Havener L. (Ed). (2008). Standards for Cancer Registries Volume III: Standards for Completeness, Quality, Analysis, and Management of Data. Springfield (IL): North American Association of Central Cancer Registries.

Holleczek B., Brenner H. (2012). Reduction of populationbased cancer survival estimates by trace back of death certificate notifications: An empirical illustration. European Journal of Cancer, 48, 797-804.

IARCcrgTools, http://www.iacr.com.fr/ (23.08.2013).

ICD-9: International statistical Classification of Diseases, revision 9 (adapted by the ministry of health; BMAGS-Version, 1989).

ICD-10: International statistical Classification of Diseases und related health problems, revision 10 http://www.dimdi.de/static/de/klassi/icd-10-who/index.htm (23.08.2013).

ICD-O-3: International Classification of Diseases for Oncology, 3rd Edition, http://www.dimdi.de/static/de/klassi/icdo3/index.htm (23.08.2013).

Jensen OM., Parkin DM., MacLennan R., Muir CS., Skeet RG. (1991). Cancer Registration: Principle and Methods, IARC Scientific Publications No. 95. Lyon: IARC.

Larsen IK., Småstuen M., Johannesen TB., Langmark F., Parkin DM., Bray F., Møller B. (2009). Data quality at the Cancer Registry of Norway: an overview of comparability completeness validity and timeliness. European Journal of Cancer, 45, 1218–31.

Leitner B. (2011). Todesursachenstatistik - Jahresergebnisse 2009; Schwerpunktthema: Sterbefälle von Personen mit Wohnsitz im Ausland. Statistische Nachrichten, 1, 34-44.

Krebsstatistikgesetz - Bundesgesetz vom 6. März 1969 über die statistische Erfassung von Geschwulstkrankheiten (Krebsstatistikgesetz [Cancer Statistics Act]) StF: BGBl. Nr. 138/1969 i.d.F. BGBl. Nr. 425/1969, http://www.ris.bka.gv.at/Dokumente/BgblPdf/1969_138_0/1969_138_0.pdf und

http://www.ris.bka.gv.at/Dokumente/BgblPdf/1969_425_0/1969_425_0.
pdf (23.08.2013).

Krebsstatistikverordnung - Verordnung des Bundesministers für Gesundheit und Umweltschutz vom 16. März 1978 über die statistische Erfassung von Geschwulstkrankheiten (Krebsstatistikverordnung [Cancer Statistics Ordinance]) StF: BGBl. Nr. 171/1978, http://www.ris.bka.gv.at/Dokumente/BgblPdf/1978_171_0/1978_171_0. pdf (23.08.2013).

Mattauch, Lehnert, Krieg und Hense. (2003).

Møller H., Richards S., Hanchett N., Riaz SP., Lüchtenborg M., Holmberg L., Robinson D. (2011). Completeness of case ascertainment and survival time error in English cancer registries: impact on 1-year survival estimates. British Journal of Cancer, 105, 170-176.

Montanaro F., Robinson D., Bordoni A. (2006). A modification to the flow method to estimate completeness in cancer registries with delayed registration. Journal of Public Health, 28, 274–7.

Muir C., Waterhouse J. (1987). Comparability and quality of data: reliability of registration. Lyon: IARC.

Oberaigner W., Concin H., Hausmanninger H. (1998). Krebsatlas Westösterreich 1988-1992, Salzburg, Tirol, Vorarlberg. Innsbruck: Eigenverlag.

Oberaigner W., Siebert U. (2009). Are survival rates for Tyrol published in the Eurocare studies biased? Acta Oncologica, 48, 984-91.

Oberaigner W., Vittadello F. (2010). Cancer mapping in alpine regions 2001-2005. Innsbruck: Eigenverlag.

Palli D. (2000). Epidemiology of gastric cancer: an evaluation of available evidence. Journal of Gastroenterology, 35 Suppl 12, 84-9.

Parkin DM., Bray F. (2009). Evaluation of data quality in the cancer registry: Principles and Methods Part II. Completeness. European Journal of Cancer, 45, 756-764.

Parkin DM., Chen VW., Ferlay J., Galceran J., Storm HH., Whealan SL. (1994). Comparability and Quality Control in Cancer Registration, IARC Technical Report No. 19. Lyon: IARC.

Parkin DM., Hakulinen T. (1991). Cancer registration: principles and methods. Analysis of survival. International Agency for Research on Cancer Scientific publication, 95, 159-76.

Parkin DM., Plummer M. (2002). Comparability and quality of data. In: Curado MP., Edwards B., Shin HR., Storm H., Ferlay J., Heanue M., Boyle P. (2007). Cancer Incidence in Five Continents Vol. IX, IARC Scientific Publication No. 160. Lyon: IARC.

Parkin DM., Whelan SL., Ferlay J., Teppo L., Thomas DB. (2002). Cancer Incidence in Five Continents Vol. VIII, IARC Scientific Publications No. 155. Lyon: IARC.

Personenstandsverordnung - Verordnung des Bundesministers für Inneres vom 14. November 1983 zur Durchführung des Personenstandsgesetzes (Personenstandsverordnung - PStV), StF: BGBl. Nr. 629/1983 i.d.F. BGBl. II Nr. 1/2010, http://www.ris.bka.gv.at/Dokument.wxe?Abfrage=BgblAuth&Dokumentnummer=BGBLA_2010_II_1 (23.08.2013).

Robert Koch Institut. (2012). Robert Koch Institut (Hrsg) und die Gesellschaft der epidemiologischen Krebsregister in Deutschland e.V. Berlin: Krebs in Deutschland 2007/2008, 8. Ausgabe. Robert Koch Institut (Hrsg.) und die Gesellschaft der epidemiologischen Krebsregister in Deutschland e.V. Berlin.

Robinson D., Use of the flow method to estimate trends in completeness of registration at the Thames Cancer Registry Cancer in South East England Cancer incidence prevalence survival and treatment for residents of South East England in 2008, http://www.thames-cancer-regorguk/informat/pubs/2008_tcr_reportpdf (14.02.2012).

Robinson D., Comp.ado—copies of the completeness software are available on request. Quoted from: Bullard J., Coleman MP., Robinson D., Lutz JM., Bell J., Peto J. (2000). Completeness of cancer registration: a new method for routine use. British Journal of Cancer, 82, 1111–16.

Robinson D., Complims.ado—copies of the completeness software are available on request. Quoted from: Bullard J., Coleman MP., Robinson D., Lutz JM., Bell J., Peto J. (2000). Completeness of cancer registration: a new method for routine use. British Journal of Cancer, 82, 1111–16.

Robinson D., Sankila R., Hakulinen T., Møller H. (2007). Interpreting international comparisons of cancer survival: The effects of incomplete registration and the presence of death certificate only cases on survival estimates. European Journal of Cancer, 43, 909-913.

SAS/STAT User's Guide [computer program]. Version 92. Cary, North Carolina: SAS Institute Inc, 2002–2008.

Schmidtmann I., Blettner M. (2009). How do cancer registries in Europe estimate completeness of registration. Methods of Information in Medicine, 48, 267-71.

Segi M. (1960). Cancer Mortality for Selected Sites in 24 Countries (1950–1957). . Sendai, Japan: Tohoku University School of Public Health.

Silcocks P. (2006). Survival of death certificate initiated registrations: selection bias, incomplete trace back or higher mortality. British Journal of Cancer, 95, 1576-8.

Silcocks P., Robinson D. (2004). Completeness of ascertainment by cancer registries: putting bounds on the number of missing cases. Journal of Public Health, 26, 161–7.

StataCorp. Stata Statistical Software [computer program]. Release 12. College Station, Texas: StataCorp LP, 2011.

Statistik Austria, http://www.statistik.at/web_de/statistiken/bevoelkerung/index.html (23.08.2013).

Statistik Austria, http://www.statistik.at/web_de/statistiken/gesundheit/krebserkrankungen/index.html (23.08.2013).

Statistik Austria: Krebsinzidenz und Krebsmortalität in Österreich 2010. (2010). Wien, Austria: Verlag Österreich GmbH.

Statistik Austria: Krebsinzidenz und Krebsmortalität in Österreich 2012. (2012). Wien, Austria: Verlag Österreich GmbH.

Statistik Austria: Jahrbuch der Gesundheitsstatistik 2009. (2010). Wien, Austria: Verlag Österreich GmbH.

Statistik Austria: Jahrbuch der Gesundheitsstatistik 2010. (2011). Wien, Austria: Verlag Österreich GmbH.

Statistik Austria: Dokumentation "Krebsstatistik", http://www.statistik.at/web_de/dokumentationen/Gesundheit/index.html (23.08.2013).

Statistik Austria: Dokumentation "Spitalsentlassungsstatistik ab 1989", http://www.statistik.at/web_de/dokumentationen/Gesundheit/index.html (23.08.2013).

Statistik Austria: Dokumentation "Statistik der Standesfälle einschließlich Todesursachenstatistik ab 2010", http://www.statistik.at/web_de/dokumentationen/Gesundheit/index.html (23.08.2013).

Vostakolaei F., Karim-Kos H., Janssen-Heijnen M., Visser O., Verbeek A., Kiemeney L. (2010). The validity of the mortality to incidence ratio as a proxy for site-specific cancer survival. European Journal of Public Health, 21, 573-7.

Waterhouse J., Muir C., Correra P., Powell J. (1976). Cancer Incidence in Five Continents Vol. III, IARC Scientific Publication No. 15. Lyon: IARC.

Zielonke N. (2011). Die Krebslast in Österreich; Berechnung der Krebsprävalenz auf Basis der Daten des österreichischen Krebsregisters. Statistische Nachrichten, 3, 187-92.

7 Glossar

Incidence .... Incidence is a measure of the risk of developing some new condition within a specified period of time. Incidence is the number of newly diagnosed cases over a specified time period. Incidence rates for cancer are mostly expressed as n/100,000 person-years.

Prevalence .... Prevalence is a measure of the burden of the disease on society. Prevalence is the proportion of the total number of cases to the total population.

Survival .... Survival percentages express the probability of surviving for a specified time period.

Mortality .... Mortality quantifies the number of cases who have died from the disease during a specified time period. Mortality rates for cancer are mostly expressed as n/100,000 person-years.

Age-specific rate .... Age-specific rates are rates for specified age groups, in which the numerator and denominator refer to the same age group.

Age-adjusted rate .... Age-adjusted rates are used to compare incidences between different regions or over time, age-adjusted rates are used.

Standard population .... Standard populations are "artificial populations" with fictitious age structures. They are used in direct aged-adjustment (age standardization) as

	uniform basis for the calculation of comparable measures for the respective reference population(s).
ENCR	European Network of Cancer Registries http://www.encr.com.fr/
IACR	International Association for Cancer Registries http://www.iacr.com.fr/
IARC	International Agency for Research on Cancer http://www.iarc.fr/
ICD-10 classification	The International Statistical Classification of Diseases and Related Health Problems (10th revision) provides a standardized coding scheme for diseases and related health problems.
ICD-O-3 classification	The International Classification of Diseases for Oncology (3rd revision) provides a standardized coding scheme for neoplasms based on localization, tumor morphology and biological behavior.
Causes of death statistics	Causes of death statistics provide information about the ultimate course of diseases in the population
Death-certificate-only (DCO) cases	DCO cases are cancer cases, which are only identified from death certificates.
Hospital discharge statistics	Hospital discharge statistics provide information about cases treated in hospitals. These statistics are based on billing data.

Hospital-discharge-only (HDO) cases ..... HDO cases are cancer cases, which are only identified from hospital discharge files.

Mortality:incidence ratio (M:I ratio) .... The Mortality:Incidence ratio (M:I ratio) is a comparison of the number of deaths and the number of new cases of a specific cancer registered in the same period of time. It is a qualitative method for completeness estimation of cancer registry data.

Flow Method .... The Flow Method, a method to estimate completeness of cancer registry data, is based on the logical flow of data in the registration system and on the time distribution of various probabilities inherent in this flow.

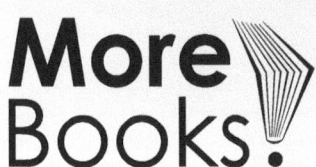
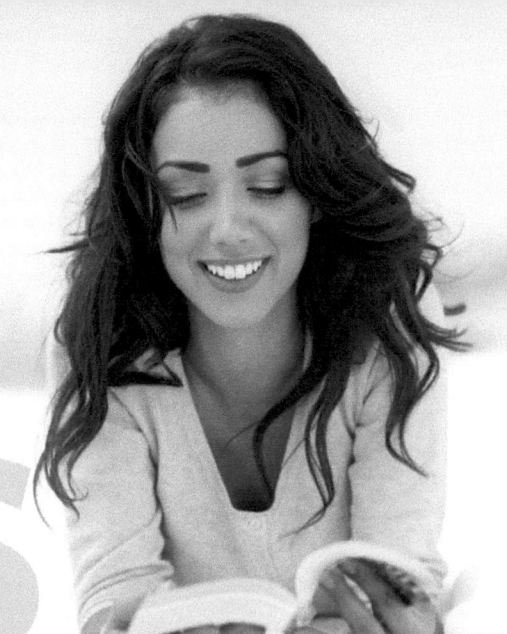

I want morebooks!

Buy your books fast and straightforward online - at one of the world's fastest growing online book stores! Environmentally sound due to Print-on-Demand technologies.

Buy your books online at
www.get-morebooks.com

Kaufen Sie Ihre Bücher schnell und unkompliziert online – auf einer der am schnellsten wachsenden Buchhandelsplattformen weltweit! Dank Print-On-Demand umwelt- und ressourcenschonend produziert.

Bücher schneller online kaufen
www.morebooks.de

VDM Verlagsservicegesellschaft mbH
Heinrich-Böcking-Str. 6-8
D - 66121 Saarbrücken   Telefax: +49 681 93 81 567-9   info@vdm-vsg.de
www.vdm-vsg.de

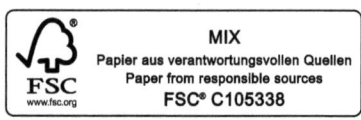

Printed by Books on Demand GmbH, Norderstedt / Germany